Easy Recipes for Health and Wellbeing

Delicious and Nutritious Dishes for a Healthy Lifestyle

BY Yannick Alcorn

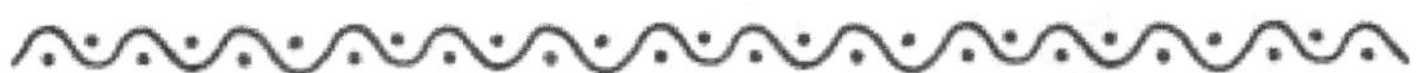

Copyright Warnings

Reproduction of this book, including photocopying, digital copying, posting on social media, printing, republishing, or selling, is prohibited without written permission from the author. Unauthorized reproductions may result in legal action.

While the author has ensured the book's authenticity and accuracy, they are not liable for any consequences arising from the reader's actions based on the information provided.

Table of Contents

Introduction

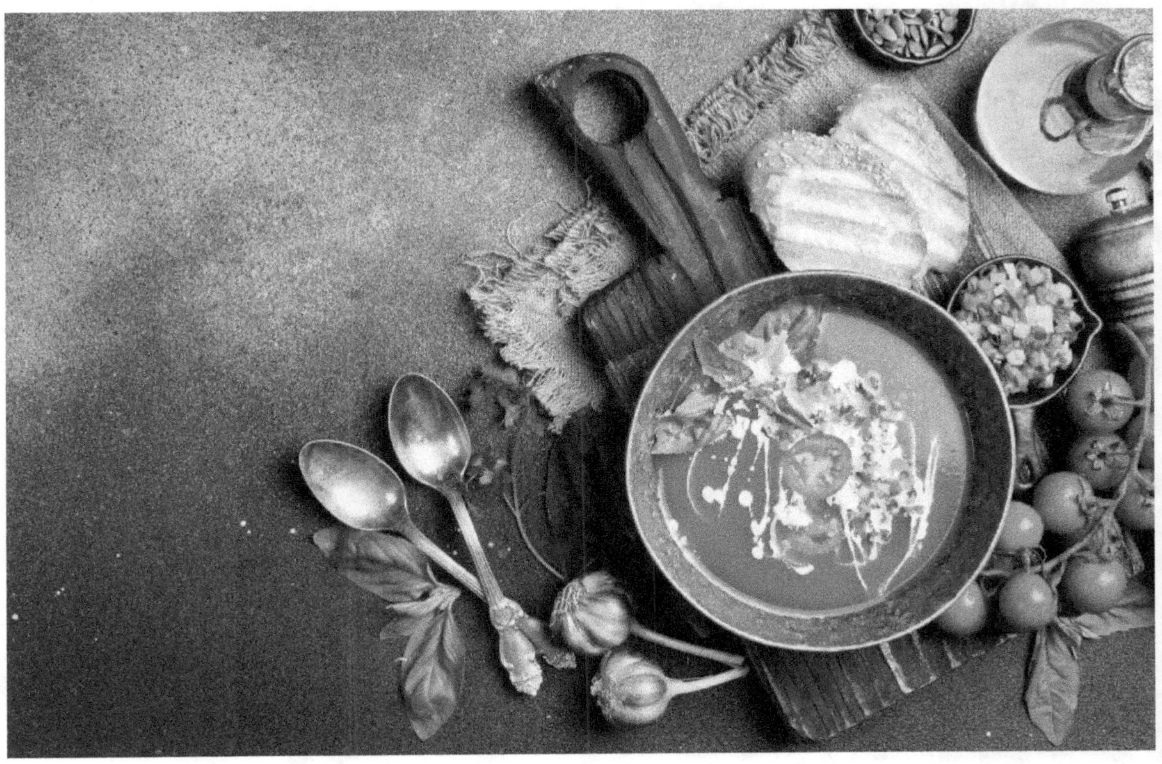

"Easy Recipes for Health and Wellbeing" is not for those seeking boring, bland "diet" food. Inside, you'll find 30 mouthwatering recipes proving healthy eating can burst with flavor.

We've developed nutritious meals so fresh and crave-worthy that you'll never feel deprived. Each recipe offers wholesome ingredients without sacrificing taste.

Explore innovative and delightful methods to fuel your body with delectable plant-based cuisine. Our creative combinations provide a rainbow of colors, textures, and flavors to keep you energized.

From savory breakfasts to hearty dinners and everything in between, these recipes make vegetables, fruits, grains and herbs the delicious stars of the plate. Food this enticing makes nutrition a reward rather than a chore.

Disprove the notion that eating light has to be boring. Our recipes transform natural, beneficial foods into craveable meals that delight the senses and taste buds.

With this cookbook, healthy eating is an adventure. Its diverse recipes will turn you into a plant-powered gourmand who relishes nutritious foods. Discover the joy of wholesome cooking you can't wait to devour.

AAAAAAAAAAAAAAAAAAAAAA

1. Ground Beef and Rice

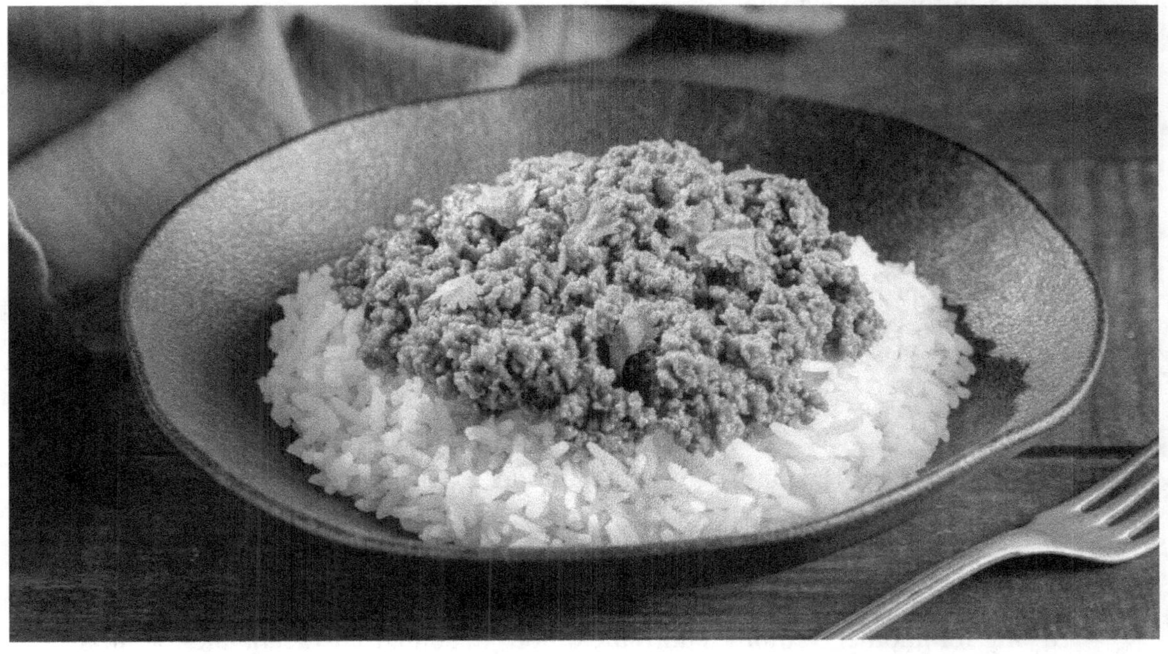

Try it out with this special Korean recipe; you'd love every bit of it!!!

Preparation Time: 06 Minutes

Cook Time: 15 Minutes

Serve: 2

List of Ingredients:

- 1 diced red bell pepper
- 2 cups of ground lean beef
- 2 tbsp of soy sauce
- 1 minced garlic clove
- 1 minced ginger
- 1 tbsp of oil

AAAAAAAAAAAAAAAAAAAAAA

Methods:

A. Heat a pan over medium-high heat and add the ground beef. Stir-fry the beef for about 4 minutes until it's browned and cooked through.

B. Toss in the chopped onion, ginger, and garlic to the cooked beef. Continue stir-frying for another 2 minutes until the onions become translucent and the mixture is fragrant.

C. Transfer the beef mixture to a plate and set it aside.

D. In the same pan, add a little oil and then put in the sliced bell pepper. Cook for about 2 minutes until it starts to soften.

E. Add the eggplant and zucchini to the pan. Continue cooking for approximately 4 minutes until the vegetables become tender.

F. Now, add honey, black pepper, vinegar, and your preferred sauce (e.g., soy sauce, teriyaki sauce, or oyster sauce) to the pan with the vegetables. Stir well to combine all the flavors.

G. Return the cooked beef to the pan and mix it with the vegetables and sauce. Let everything cook together for a couple of minutes to allow the flavors to meld.

H. Once everything is heated through and well-cooked, your Ground Beef and Rice is ready to be served.

I. Serve the dish over a bed of cooked rice, and garnish it with chopped green onions for a fresh and vibrant touch.

Cooking Notes:

A. For the ground beef, choose a leaner option to avoid excess grease in the dish.

B. Make sure to break up the ground beef while cooking to ensure even cooking and avoid large clumps.

C. You can adjust the cooking time for the vegetables based on your desired level of tenderness. Some prefer their veggies slightly crisp, while others like them softer.

D. Feel free to add more vegetables or substitute with your favorites, such as carrots, broccoli, or snow peas.

E. The choice of sauce will greatly impact the flavor of the dish. Experiment with different sauces to find the one you like best.

F. Be cautious with the amount of honey and vinegar used. Adjust according to your preference for sweetness and tanginess.

G. Taste the dish before serving and add a pinch of salt if needed, but be mindful of the salt content in the chosen sauce.

H. If you like some heat, you can add crushed red pepper flakes or sliced chili peppers during the cooking process.

I. The dish can also be served with noodles instead of rice if preferred.

2. Green Apple Juice

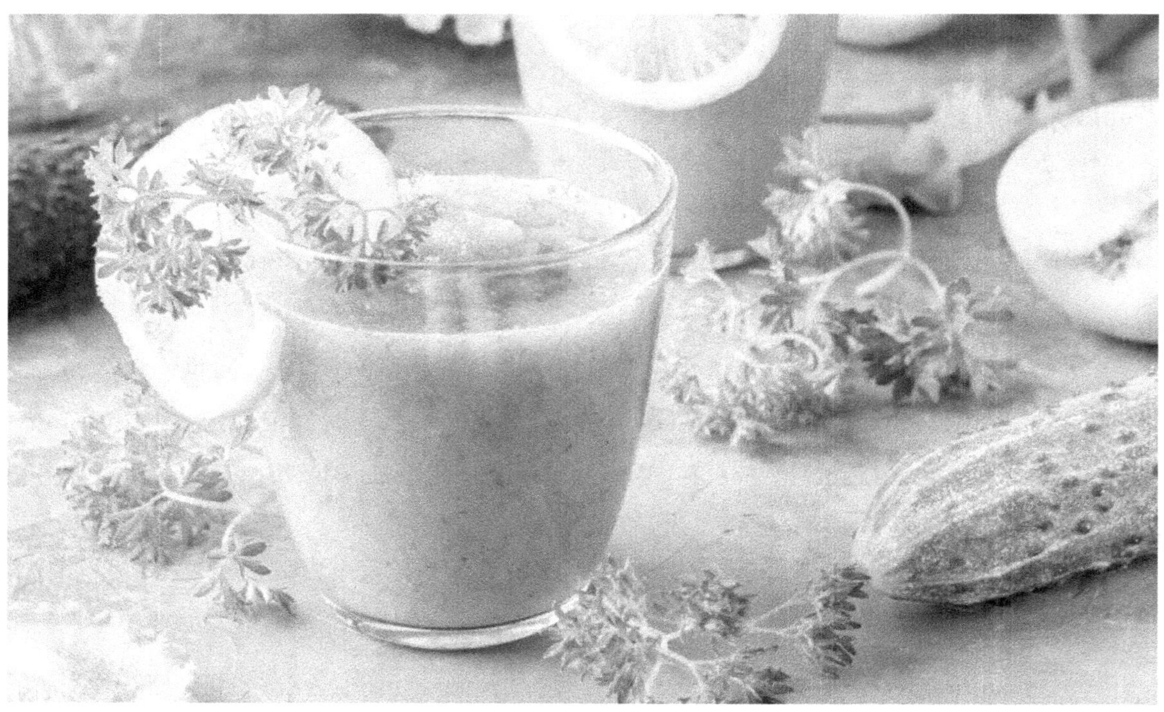

Something blissful, delicious and healthy for hot summer days!!

Preparation Time: 03 Minutes

Cook Time: Nil

Serve: 2

List of Ingredients:

- 2 cored green apples (chopped)
- 1 chopped cucumber
- 1 ginger
- 6 celery stalks

AAAAAAAAAAAAAAAAAAAAAA

Methods:

A. Prepare the ingredients by coring and chopping 2 green apples, chopping 1 cucumber, and peeling a small piece of ginger.
B. Put the cored green apples, chopped cucumber, ginger, and 6 celery stalks into a food processor.
C. Process the ingredients in the food processor until you achieve the desired consistency of the juice.
D. Once the Green Apple Juice is ready, serve it immediately.
E. Enjoy your refreshing and nutritious Green Apple Juice.

Cooking Notes:

A. Choosing fresh and ripe green apples will ensure a sweet and flavorful juice. Feel free to mix different varieties of green apples for a more complex taste.
B. Cucumbers add a subtle, refreshing taste to the juice, but make sure they are fresh and not bitter.
C. Ginger adds a hint of spiciness and warmth to the juice. Adjust the quantity based on your preference for the intensity of ginger flavor.
D. Celery stalks provide a slightly salty and herbal taste, balancing the sweetness of the apples and the freshness of the cucumber.

E. You can add a squeeze of lemon juice to enhance the brightness and tanginess of the juice.

F. If you prefer a thinner consistency, you can strain the juice through a fine mesh sieve or nut milk bag after processing.

G. For a cooler and more refreshing juice, you can add a few ice cubes to the food processor before processing the ingredients.

H. If you don't have a food processor, you can use a blender instead. However, keep in mind that using a blender may require a little water to help with blending.

I. Experiment with the ingredient ratios to suit your taste preferences. You can add more apples for a sweeter juice or adjust the amount of cucumber and celery for a more herbal and earthy flavor.

J. Green Apple Juice is best consumed fresh to retain its nutrients and vibrant taste. If you have leftover juice, store it in an airtight container in the refrigerator and consume it within a day for the best quality. Shake well before drinking, as separation may occur over time.

3. Papaya and Yogurt Smoothie

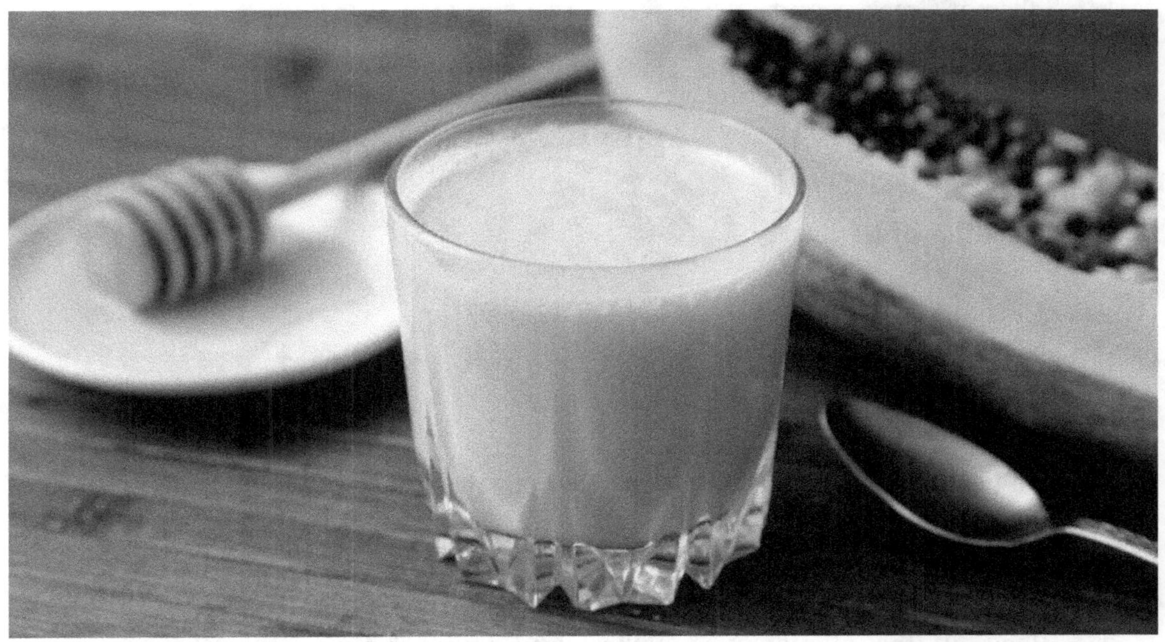

Papaya and yogurt combined with agave nectar make this smoothie one of the most surprising smoothie combos you can think of.

Preparation Time: 03 Minutes

Cook Time: Nil

Serve: 1

List of Ingredients:

- 1 tbsp of agave nectar
- 8 tbsp of Greek yogurt
- 1 handful of mint leaves
- 1 cup of chopped papaya
- 1 tbsp of lemon juice
- 2 handfuls of ice

AAAAAAAAAAAAAAAAAAAAAA

Methods:

A. In a blender, combine 1 cup of chopped papaya, 8 tbsp of Greek yogurt, 1 tbsp of agave nectar, 1 tbsp of lemon juice, and 1 handful of mint leaves.

B. Add 2 handfuls of ice to the blender to make the smoothie chilled and refreshing.

C. Blend all the ingredients together until you achieve a smooth and creamy consistency.

D. Once the Papaya and Yogurt Smoothie is well blended, pour it into glasses and serve immediately.

Cooking Notes:

A. Use ripe and sweet papaya for the smoothie to ensure a naturally sweet taste. Adjust the amount of agave nectar according to your preference for sweetness.

B. Greek yogurt provides a creamy and thick texture to the smoothie. You can use plain regular yogurt if Greek yogurt is not available, but the smoothie may be slightly less creamy.

C. Mint leaves add a fresh and aromatic element to the smoothie. You can adjust the quantity of mint leaves based on how strong you want the mint flavor to be.

D. If you want a thinner consistency, you can add a splash of milk or water while blending. Conversely, if you prefer a thicker smoothie, reduce the amount of liquid.

E. Adding lemon juice not only enhances the flavor but also helps balance the sweetness of the papaya and agave nectar.

F. Make sure to blend the smoothie until all the ingredients are well combined and there are no large chunks of papaya or mint leaves remaining.

G. If you don't have agave nectar, you can use honey or maple syrup as a natural sweetener alternative.

H. For a creamier and richer smoothie, you can add a small banana or a scoop of frozen yogurt or ice cream to the mix.

I. Feel free to customize the smoothie with additional ingredients like chia seeds, flaxseeds, or protein powder to boost its nutritional value.

J. If you prefer a dairy-free version, you can use plant-based yogurt like almond, soy, or coconut yogurt instead of Greek yogurt.

K. Serve the smoothie immediately to enjoy its fresh taste and vibrant color. If you have leftovers, store them in the refrigerator and give the smoothie a good shake before consuming, as separation may occur over time.

4. Chicken Breast and Tomatoes

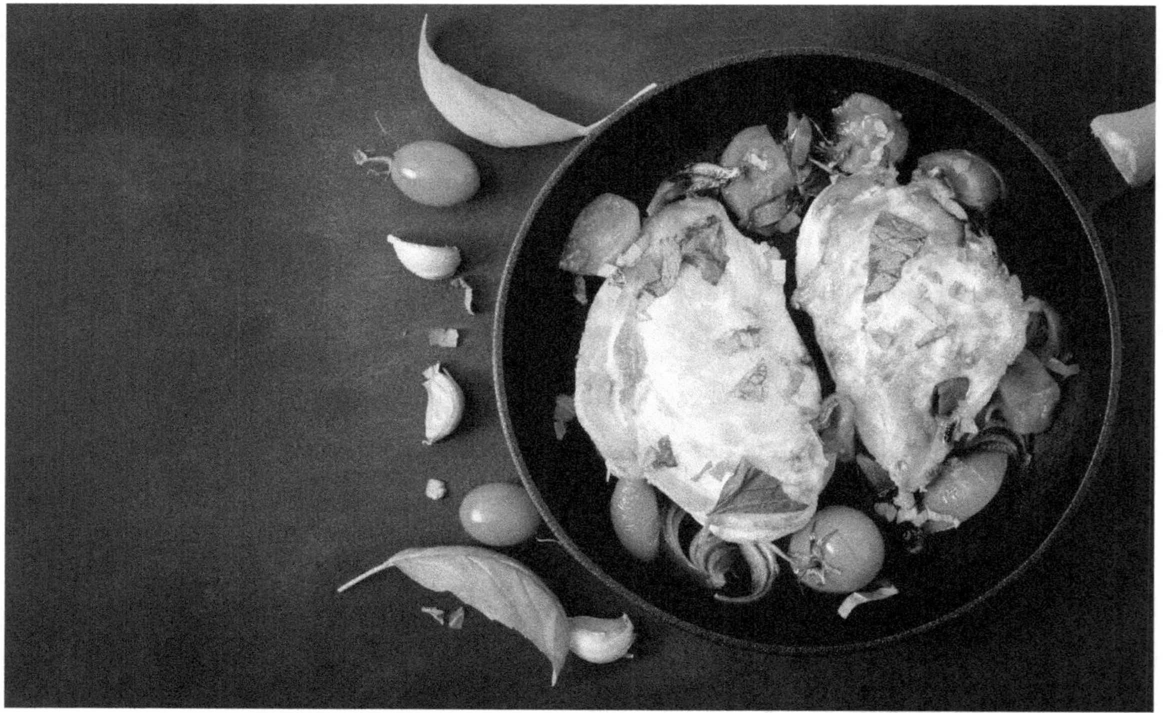

It is definitely the best chicken and tomatoes recipe you have ever tried!!

Preparation Time: 05 Minutes

Cook Time: 12 Minutes

Serve: 4

List of Ingredients:

- 1 tbsp of pepper
- 1 lb. of lean chicken breast (chunked)
- 1 tbsp of salt
- 1 tbsp of oil
- 1 pinch of dried oregano

For the Sauce:

- 3 minced garlic cloves
- 1 tbsp of pepper
- 1 handful of chopped basil
- 1 pinch of salt
- 2 large-sized ripe tomatoes
- 1 pinch of dried oregano

AAAAAAAAAAAAAAAAAAAAAAA

Methods:

A. In a bowl, combine the chicken breast pieces with salt, pepper, and oregano, tossing them well to evenly coat the chicken.
B. Heat oil in a pan and sauté the seasoned chicken pieces until they are fully cooked and browned on both sides. Once cooked, transfer the chicken to a separate plate.
C. In the same pan, add the tomatoes and the remaining sauce ingredients, along with 1 tbsp of oil. Cook until the tomatoes start to pop and release their juices.
D. Return the cooked chicken to the pan and add fresh basil for added flavor.

E. The Chicken Breast and Tomatoes dish is now ready to be served, and it goes well with rice.

Cooking Notes:

A. For the chicken breasts, you can use boneless, skinless chicken breasts for a healthier option. You can also use chicken thighs or any other preferred part of the chicken.

B. When sautéing the chicken, make sure the pan is hot enough to sear the chicken and create a nice crust on the outside. This helps to seal in the juices and keep the chicken tender and moist on the inside.

C. Avoid overcrowding the pan while sautéing the chicken, as overcrowding can cause the chicken to steam rather than brown. Cook the chicken in batches if needed.

D. If you want a richer flavor, you can marinate the chicken in the salt, pepper, oregano, and a little olive oil for 30 minutes to an hour before cooking. This will help infuse the chicken with the herb and spice flavors.

E. When cooking the tomatoes, use ripe and flavorful tomatoes for the best results. Cherry or grape tomatoes work well in this dish as they hold their shape and have a slightly sweeter taste.

F. If the tomatoes are not releasing enough juices while cooking, you can add a splash of chicken broth or water to help create a sauce.

G. The fresh basil adds a burst of herbal aroma and flavor to the dish. You can tear the basil leaves or chop them, depending on your preference.

H. Feel free to add other vegetables to the dish, such as bell peppers, zucchini, or spinach, to make it more colorful and nutritious.

I. To serve, you can plate the Chicken Breast and Tomatoes over cooked rice or pasta, or alongside some crusty bread to soak up the flavorful tomato sauce.

5. Chicken, Corn and Zucchini

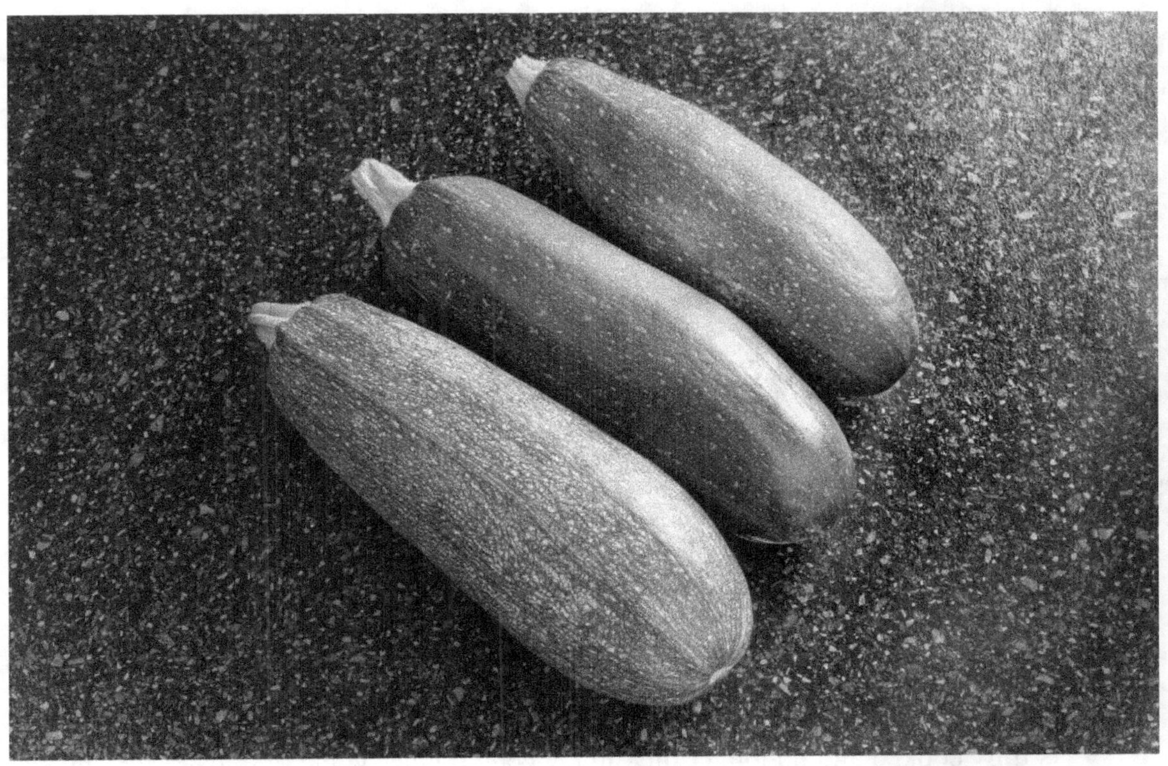

A pan of awesome deliciousness!!!

Preparation Time: 05 Minutes

Cook Time: 15 Minutes

Serve: 2

List of Ingredients:

- 2 tbsp of pepper
- 1 tbsp of salt
- 2 pounds of lean chicken breast (cut into pieces)
- 2 tbsp of canola oil
- 1 lb. of zucchini
- 1 cup of corn
- 1 minced garlic clove
- 1 cup of chopped parsley

AAAAAAAAAAAAAAAAAAAAAAAA

Methods:

A. Cut the zucchini into half-moon slices to prepare it for cooking.

B. In a skillet, sauté garlic in oil for about 3 minutes to release its flavor and aroma.

C. Add the chicken to the skillet along with salt and pepper. Cook the chicken until it is fully cooked and no longer pink in the center. Once cooked, transfer the chicken to a separate plate.

D. In the same skillet, add the zucchini, corn, salt, and pepper. Cook the vegetables for approximately 4 minutes until they become tender.

E. Return the cooked chicken to the skillet with the zucchini and corn mixture.

F. Toss the ingredients together in the skillet to combine all the flavors.

G. Serve the Chicken, Corn, and Zucchini over a bed of rice and garnish it with fresh parsley for a burst of color and added freshness.

H. Enjoy this delicious and nutritious dish with the delightful combination of chicken, corn, and zucchini.

Cooking Notes:

A. To cut the zucchini into half-moon slices, slice it vertically first, then lay each half flat on the cutting board and slice diagonally into semi-circular pieces.

B. When sautéing the garlic in oil, make sure not to burn it, as burnt garlic can become bitter. Cook it over medium heat until it becomes fragrant and slightly golden.

C. For the chicken, you can use boneless, skinless chicken breasts or chicken thighs. Cut the chicken into bite-sized pieces for even and quick cooking.

D. Season the chicken with salt and pepper to enhance its flavor. You can also add other spices or herbs, such as paprika or thyme, for additional taste.

E. When cooking the chicken, avoid overcooking it, as this can lead to dry and tough meat. Remove it from the skillet as soon as it is fully cooked and transfer it to a plate to keep it juicy.

F. For the zucchini and corn, cooking them for a few minutes ensures they remain crisp and retain their natural sweetness.

G. The dish can be customized with other vegetables like bell peppers, cherry tomatoes, or broccoli, depending on personal preferences.

H. For added creaminess, you can stir in a bit of heavy cream or grated cheese to the skillet before serving.

I. Serve the Chicken, Corn, and Zucchini mixture over any type of rice you prefer, such as white rice, brown rice, or quinoa, to create a balanced and satisfying meal.

J. Leftovers can be refrigerated and reheated for another meal. However, the vegetables may become slightly softer upon reheating.

K. Feel free to adjust the seasonings and ingredients according to your taste and dietary preferences.

6. Cauliflower Fried Rice

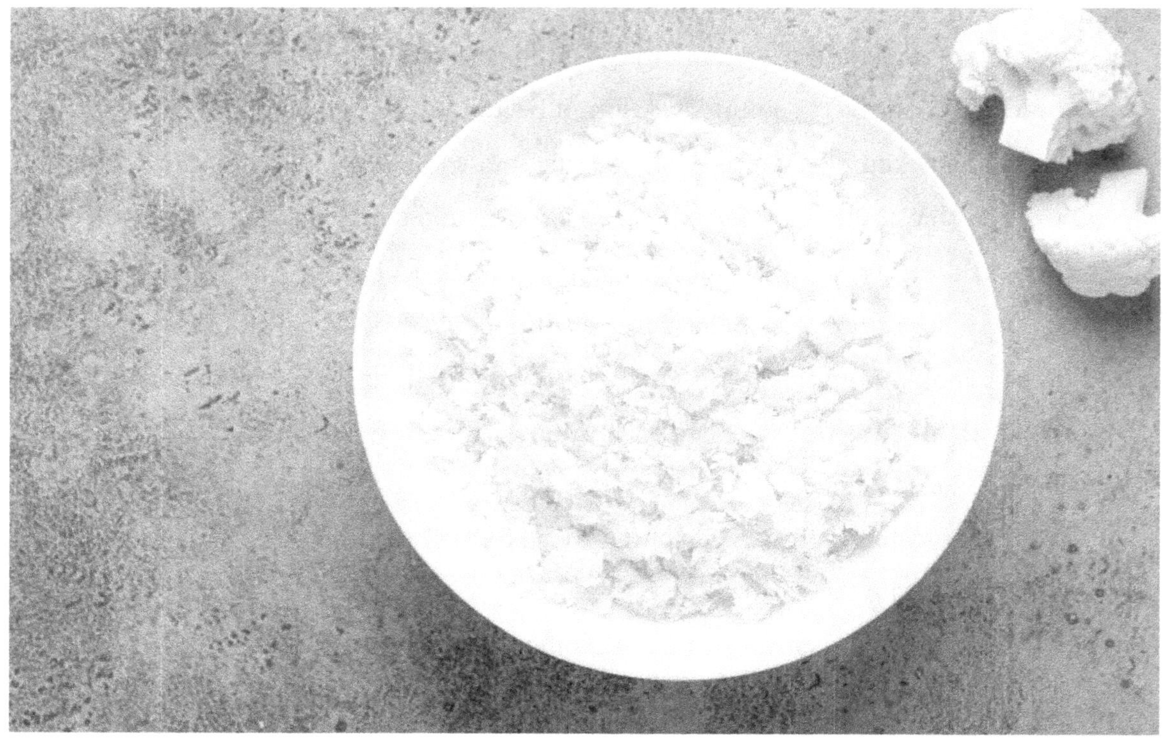

You know when you have curry in a stir-fry meal, the meal is about to blow your palate away!!

Preparation Time: 03 Minutes

Cook Time: 10 Minutes

Serve: 2

List of Ingredients:

- 2 handfuls of peas
- 1 chopped onion
- 2 large-sized eggs (beaten)
- 1 chopped onion sprig
- 1 tbsp of maple syrup
- 7 oz of cauliflower rice
- 1 diced medium-sized carrot
- 1 tsp of minced ginger
- 1 tsp of minced garlic
- 1 tbsp of sesame oil (toasted)
- 2 tbsp of soy sauce

AAAAAAAAAAAAAAAAAAAAAAA

Methods:

A. In a pan with oil, sauté ginger, onion, garlic, peas, and carrot together.

B. Cook the mixture for about 3 minutes until the vegetables become tender and fragrant.

C. Push the vegetable mixture to one side of the pan, and crack an egg on the other side.

D. Scramble the egg for approximately 2 minutes until it's fully cooked.

E. Add the cauliflower to the pan, mixing it with the cooked vegetables and egg.

F. Toss everything together to combine the flavors and ensure even distribution of the ingredients.

G. Create space on one side of the pan again, and add the sauce and honey to that space.

H. Toss the cauliflower fried rice in the sauce and honey, making sure it coats the mixture evenly.

I. Garnish the dish with chopped green onions for a fresh and colorful touch.

J. Serve the delicious Cauliflower Fried Rice and enjoy its healthy and flavorful goodness.

Cooking Notes:

A. You can use fresh or frozen vegetables for this recipe. If using frozen peas and carrots, make sure to thaw them before cooking.

B. When sautéing the ginger, onion, garlic, peas, and carrots, be mindful not to overcook them. They should be tender but still have a slight crunch for texture.

C. For the cauliflower, you can use fresh cauliflower florets and pulse them in a food processor until they resemble rice-like grains. Alternatively, you can use store-bought cauliflower rice.

D. The egg adds protein and a nice texture to the fried rice. Scrambling the egg separately and then mixing it with the vegetables ensures even distribution throughout the dish.

E. The sauce can be a combination of soy sauce, oyster sauce, or any other preferred stir-fry sauce. Adjust the amount of sauce to your taste preference for saltiness and umami flavor.

F. The honey adds a touch of sweetness to balance the savory flavors of the dish. You can adjust the amount of honey based on your desired level of sweetness.

G. Feel free to add other vegetables or protein sources like broccoli, bell peppers, chicken, or shrimp to make the dish more nutritious and satisfying.

H. If you like your cauliflower fried rice spicier, you can add some crushed red pepper flakes or sliced chili peppers during the cooking process.

I. To keep the dish low-carb and gluten-free, use gluten-free soy sauce or tamari and check the ingredients of the stir-fry sauce for any gluten-containing additives.

J. Cauliflower fried rice is a versatile dish that can be customized to suit your dietary preferences and taste buds. Feel free to experiment with different vegetables, sauces, and seasonings to create your perfect version.

7. Chicken and Vegetable Stir Fry

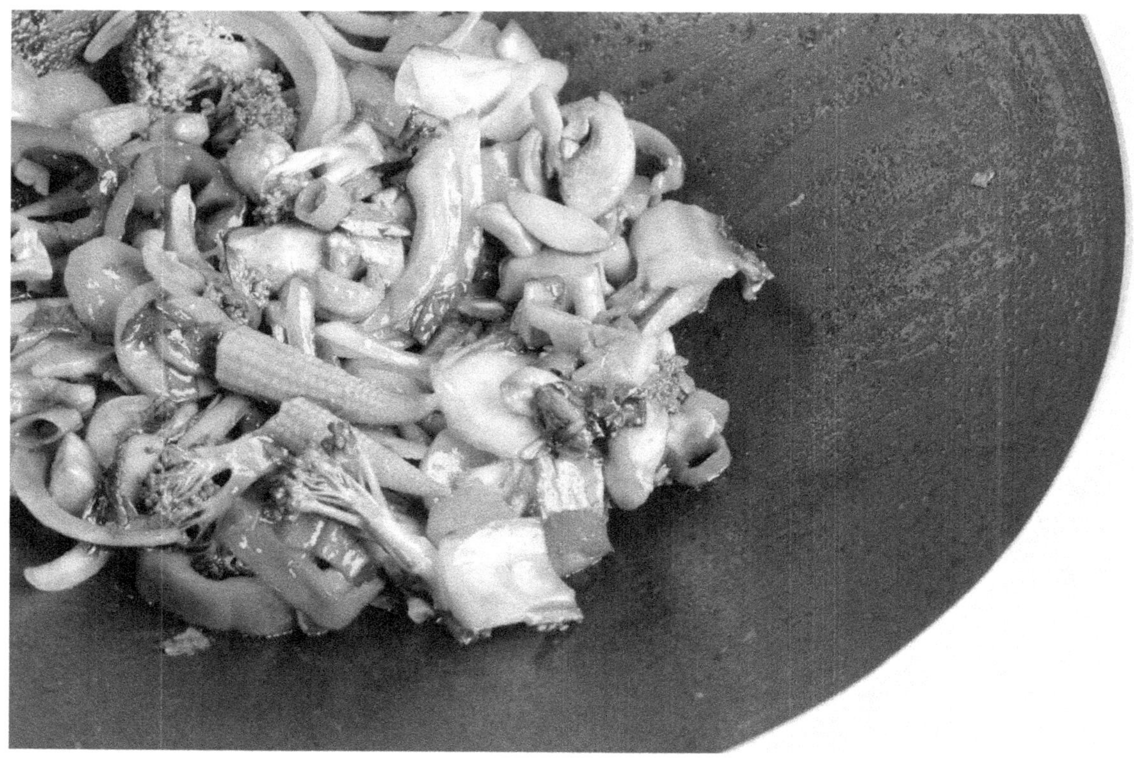

It Tastes better than what you are used to!

Preparation Time: 04 Minutes

Cook Time: 13 Minutes

Serve: 2

List of Ingredients:

- 1 chopped garlic clove
- 1 chopped broccolini
- 120g of sliced mushrooms
- 1 sliced chili (deseeded)
- 1 tbsp of soy sauce
- 1 piece of chopped ginger
- 1 sliced capsicum
- 2 lean chicken breasts (cut into strips)
- 1 chopped brown onion
- 2 tbsp of canola oil
- 1 tsp of water
- 1 tbsp of oyster sauce

AAAAAAAAAAAAAAAAAAAAAA

Methods:

A. Sauté the chicken in a pan with oil until it's fully cooked. Then, transfer the cooked chicken to a bowl.

B. In the same pan, add another tablespoon of oil and stir-fry the capsicum and onion for about 2 minutes until they become tender and slightly caramelized.

C. Add the ginger, salt, broccolini, mushrooms, chili, and garlic to the pan. Continue to cook and stir the mixture for approximately 5 minutes until the vegetables are crisp-tender.

D. Toss in water and sauces (such as soy sauce or oyster sauce) and cook for an additional minute to create a savory and flavorful sauce.

E. Return the cooked chicken to the pan and cook everything together for about 4 minutes, allowing the flavors to meld.

F. Once the Chicken and Vegetable Stir Fry is ready, serve it with rice and garnish it with fresh coriander leaves for added freshness and aroma.

Cooking Notes:

A. For the chicken, you can use boneless, skinless chicken breasts or chicken thighs, cut into bite-sized pieces. Ensure that the chicken is fully cooked and no longer pink in the center before transferring it to the bowl.

B. When sautéing the capsicum and onion, cook them over medium-high heat to develop a slight char and enhance their natural sweetness.

C. Broccolini is a hybrid vegetable, a cross between broccoli and Chinese kale. If you can't find broccolini, regular broccoli florets can be used as a substitute.

D. For the chili, you can use any type you prefer, such as red chili flakes, sliced fresh chili peppers, or chili sauce. Adjust the amount of chili according to your desired level of spiciness.

E. The sauce can be a combination of soy sauce, oyster sauce, or any other stir-fry sauce you like. Be cautious with adding extra salt, as soy sauce and other sauces can be quite salty on their own.

F. If the pan becomes too dry during cooking, you can add a splash of water or chicken broth to prevent the ingredients from sticking to the pan.

G. Make sure to cook the vegetables until they are tender but still retain some crunch for texture and color.

H. For a more nutritious stir-fry, consider adding other vegetables such as carrots, snap peas, baby corn, or bamboo shoots.

I. Feel free to customize the stir-fry with additional seasonings or spices to suit your taste preferences. You can also add a splash of sesame oil at the end for extra nutty flavor.

J. Serve the Chicken and Vegetable Stir Fry with steamed white or brown rice, or even noodles for a complete and satisfying meal. You can also pair it with quinoa or cauliflower rice for a low-carb option.

8. Cilantro and Celery Juice Punch

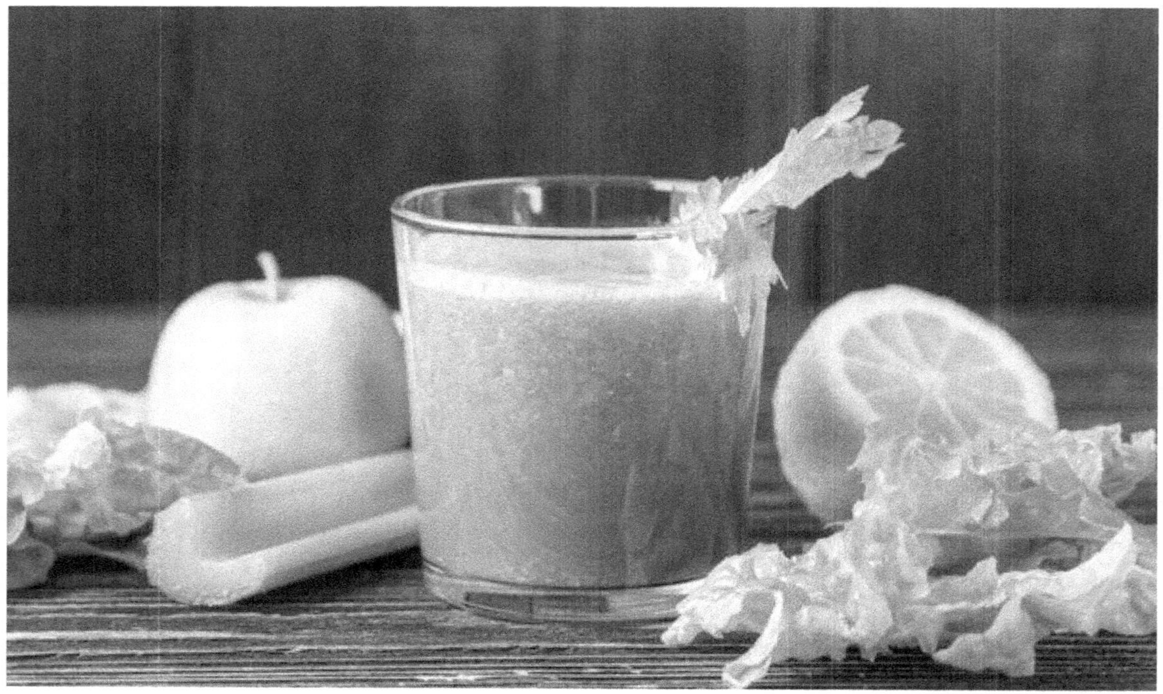

Dear cilantro lovers, this glass of richness is all yours!!!

Preparation Time: 04 Minutes

Cook Time: Nil

Serve: 1

List of Ingredients:

- 1 cored apple
- 1 ginger
- 5 celery ribs
- 3 oz of cilantro
- 2 tbsp of lemon juice

AAAAAAAAAAAAAAAAAAAAAA

Methods:

A. Juice the cored apple, ginger, celery ribs, and cilantro in a juicer to extract their fresh flavors and nutrients.
B. After juicing the other ingredients, add the lemon juice to the mixture and give it a good stir to enhance the overall taste.
C. Serve the refreshing Cilantro and Celery Juice Punch and savor its vibrant and invigorating combination of flavors.

Cooking Notes:

A. Cilantro and Celery Juice Punch is a nutritious and refreshing beverage that provides a boost of vitamins and antioxidants.
B. When juicing the apple, make sure to remove the core and seeds, as they can add bitterness to the juice.
C. Ginger adds a zingy and warming flavor to the juice. Adjust the amount of ginger based on your preference for spiciness.
D. Celery ribs are crunchy and bring a mild, earthy taste to the juice. Select fresh and crisp celery for the best results.

E. Cilantro, also known as coriander leaves, contributes a bright and herbaceous note to the juice. You can adjust the amount of cilantro to your liking.

F. Lemon juice adds a tangy and citrusy kick to balance the sweetness of the apple and the earthiness of the other ingredients.

G. To extract the most juice from the ingredients, use a high-quality juicer. If you don't have a juicer, you can use a blender and strain the juice through a fine-mesh sieve or a nut milk bag to remove any pulp.

H. Consider using organic fruits and vegetables when possible to reduce exposure to pesticides and chemicals.

I. The Cilantro and Celery Juice Punch is best served fresh to preserve its vibrant flavors and nutritional value. However, you can store any leftover juice in the refrigerator for a day or two. Just make sure to give it a good stir before serving, as natural separation may occur.

J. If you prefer a sweeter juice, you can add a small amount of honey or agave nectar. Alternatively, for a bit of extra zing, you can add a pinch of salt or a dash of cayenne pepper.

K. Feel free to customize the juice punch to suit your taste preferences. You can add other fruits or vegetables such as cucumber, spinach, or pineapple for additional flavors and nutrients.

L. Cilantro and Celery Juice Punch is a great way to incorporate more greens into your diet and boost your overall health and well-being. Enjoy it as a morning pick-me-up or as a refreshing beverage throughout the day.

9. Kiwi and Spinach Smoothie

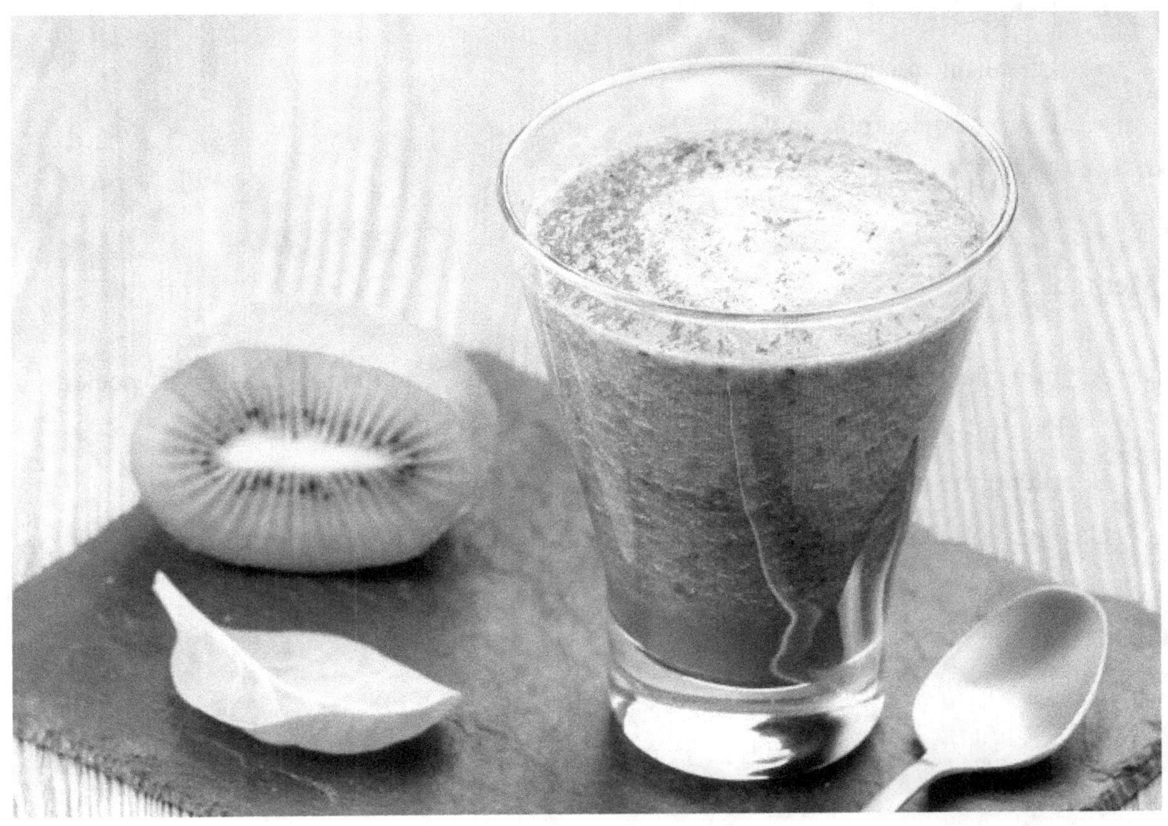

A glass of energy-boosting ingredients!!

Preparation Time: 05 Minutes

Cook Time: Nil

Serve: 1

List of Ingredients:

- 6 tbsp of coconut water
- 1 chopped kiwi fruit (peeled)
- 1 handful of chopped spinach
- 1 cup of diced pineapple

AAAAAAAAAAAAAAAAAAAAAAAA

Methods:

A. In a blender, combine 6 tbsp of coconut water, 1 chopped kiwi fruit (peeled), 1 handful of chopped spinach, and 1 cup of diced pineapple.
B. Blend the ingredients until you achieve a smooth and creamy consistency.
C. Pour the Kiwi and Spinach Smoothie into glasses and serve immediately.

Cooking Notes:

A. For a creamier texture, you can add some Greek yogurt or a frozen banana to the blender along with the other ingredients.

B. If you prefer a sweeter smoothie, consider adding a drizzle of honey or a few dates to enhance the sweetness without compromising on healthiness.

C. To make the smoothie colder and more refreshing, you can use frozen kiwi, pineapple, or spinach. Alternatively, you can add some ice cubes to the blender before blending.

D. For a protein boost, consider adding a scoop of your favorite protein powder or some chia seeds to the smoothie. This can make it a more satisfying and nutritious drink, especially if you're having it as a meal replacement.

E. If you find the smoothie too thick, you can dilute it with a bit more coconut water or regular water until you reach your desired consistency.

F. This smoothie is best consumed immediately after blending to retain the vibrant color and optimal taste. However, if you have leftovers, you can store them in an airtight container in the refrigerator for up to 24 hours. Shake well before drinking as natural separation may occur. Avoid storing it for an extended period as the freshness and nutrients may diminish.

10. Thai Salmon

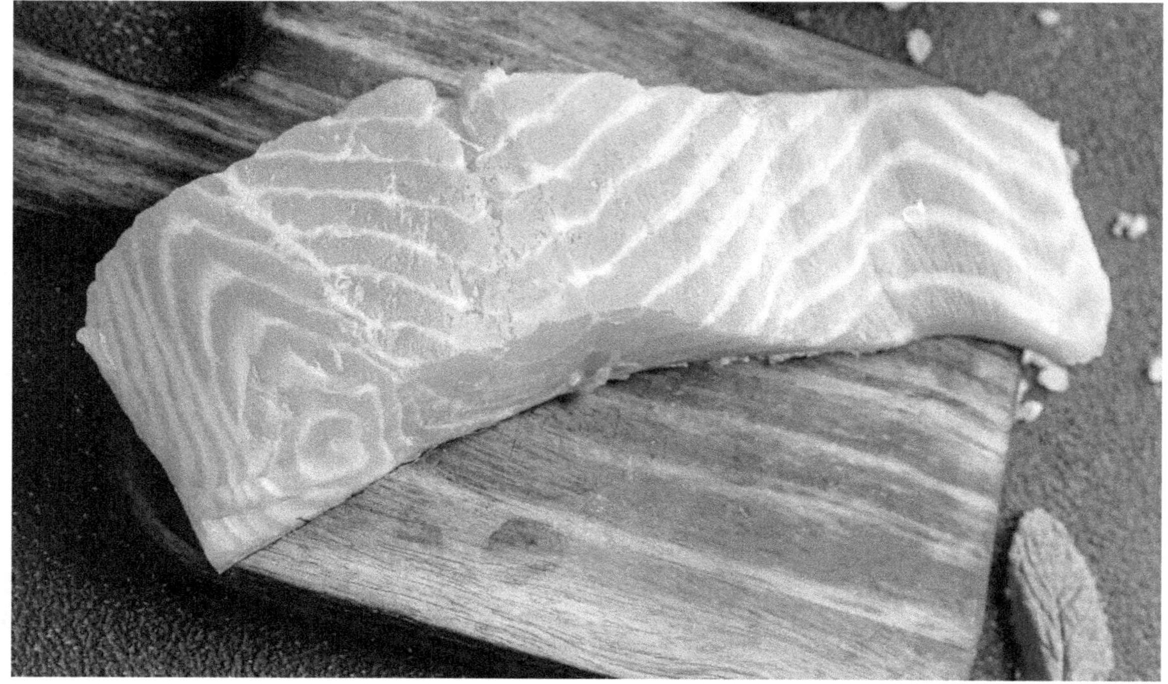

Exotic and quick can be used in the same sentence with this meal!!

Preparation Time: 10 Minutes

Cook Time: 15 Minutes

Serve: 4

List of Ingredients:

- 2 minced garlic cloves
- 4 salmon filets
- 2 tbsp of soy sauce
- 2 tbsp of lemon juice
- 1 cup of Thai chili sauce
- 1 bunch of chopped coriander
- 2 tbsp of oil
- 1 tbsp of fish sauce
- 1 tbsp of minced ginger
- 1 cup of chopped peanuts

AAAAAAAAAAAAAAAAAAAAAAA

Methods:

A. Season the salmon with your choice of seasonings, such as salt, pepper, and any other preferred herbs or spices.

B. Heat some oil in a pan and fry the marinated salmon pieces, making sure to cook both sides until the salmon is fully cooked and nicely browned.

C. Once the salmon is cooked, transfer it to a plate and set it aside.

D. In the same pan, add more oil if needed, and sauté the ginger and garlic for about 2 minutes until they become fragrant.

E. Pour in the sauces (Thai sauces like soy sauce, fish sauce, or oyster sauce) and lemon juice into the pan with the ginger and garlic. Stir the mixture for another 2 minutes, allowing the flavors to meld together.

F. Now, serve the cooked salmon on a plate and drizzle the sauce you prepared in the pan over the salmon.

G. Garnish the dish with fresh coriander (cilantro) and chopped peanuts to add extra flavor and texture.

H. Your Thai Salmon is ready to be enjoyed!

Cooking Notes:

A. For seasoning the salmon, you can get creative and use various herbs and spices like paprika, cumin, or chili powder to add depth to the flavor. Thai-inspired seasonings like lemongrass, lime zest, or Thai red curry paste can also be excellent choices.

B. When frying the salmon, make sure the oil is hot enough before placing the salmon in the pan. This will help create a nice sear on the outside while keeping the inside moist and tender. Don't overcrowd the pan; cook the salmon in batches if necessary.

C. To prevent the salmon from sticking to the pan, use a non-stick pan or make sure to oil the pan adequately before frying.

D. Thai sauces like soy sauce, fish sauce, and oyster sauce are rich and flavorful. Adjust the quantities of these sauces based on your taste preferences and dietary restrictions.

E. For added freshness and tanginess, you can squeeze some lime juice over the salmon before serving.

F. If you prefer a spicier dish, you can add sliced Thai red chilies or chili flakes to the sauce during the sautéing process.

G. Serve the Thai Salmon with steamed rice or noodles to make it a complete and satisfying meal.

H. Feel free to customize the garnishes as well. Besides coriander and peanuts, you can use sliced green onions, toasted sesame seeds, or thinly sliced red bell peppers to add color and crunch to the dish.

11. Spiced Crunchy Salad

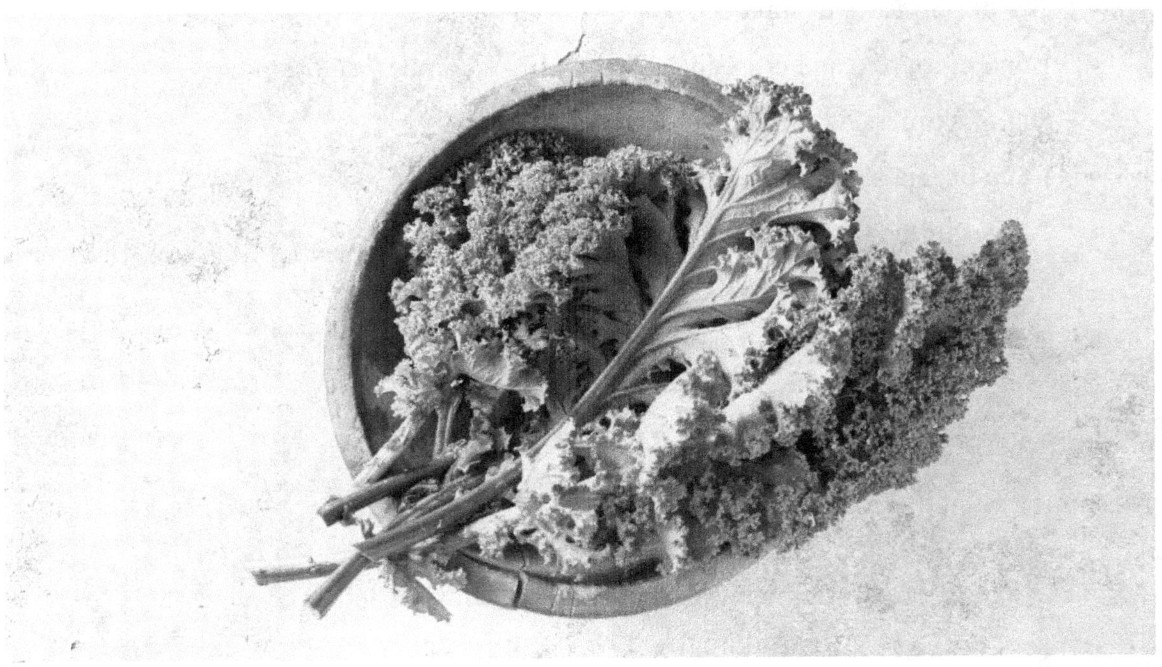

Salad has never tasted this healthy and crunchy!!

Preparation Time: 07 Minutes

Cook Time: Nil

Serve: 3

List of Ingredients:

- 1 sliced head of broccoli (toasted)
- 80g of purple kale (shredded)
- 1 cup of toasted and crushed seeds (cumin, coriander, and sesame)
- 50g of skinless hazelnuts (crushed)
- 1 cup of feta and mustard dressing
- 2 slices of ciabatta (toasted and shredded)
- 1 sliced small cauliflower
- 80g of chopped spinach leaves

AAAAAAAAAAAAAAAAAAAAAAAA

Methods:

A. In a large bowl, combine fresh spinach, cauliflower, and kale.
B. Toss the vegetables well to mix them evenly.
C. Add diced ciabatta bread and broccoli into the bowl and mix again.
D. Garnish the salad with your preferred dressing, seeds (such as sesame or sunflower seeds), and nuts (like almonds or walnuts).

Cooking Notes:

A. For the dressing, you can use a variety of options. A simple vinaigrette made with olive oil, balsamic vinegar, Dijon mustard, salt, and pepper would work well. Alternatively, you can use a creamy dressing like Caesar or ranch for a richer flavor.

B. If using raw cauliflower and broccoli, you can blanch or steam them for a few minutes before adding them to the salad. This will soften them slightly and make them easier to chew while retaining their crispiness.

C. For added protein, you can include some grilled chicken, tofu, or chickpeas in the salad.

D. You can also add other vegetables or fruits of your choice, such as cherry tomatoes, cucumbers, bell peppers, or diced apples, to enhance the salad's flavor and texture.

E. To make it more filling and satisfying as a main dish, you can add some cooked quinoa or couscous to the salad.

F. If you prefer a warm salad, you can lightly sauté the spinach, cauliflower, kale, and broccoli before mixing them with the other ingredients. The warm vegetables will slightly wilt the greens and add a comforting touch to the dish.

G. Feel free to experiment with different herbs and spices to enhance the flavors. Fresh herbs like basil, cilantro, or mint can add a burst of freshness to the salad.

H. To keep the ciabatta bread crunchy, it's best to add it just before serving. If you let it sit in the dressing for too long, it may become soggy.

I. For a more tangy and zesty taste, you can add a squeeze of lemon or lime juice to the salad before tossing. The citrusy flavor will brighten up the dish.

J. Remember to adjust the seasoning according to your taste preferences. You can add more salt, pepper, or other spices to suit your liking.

12. Tomato Kale Gazpacho

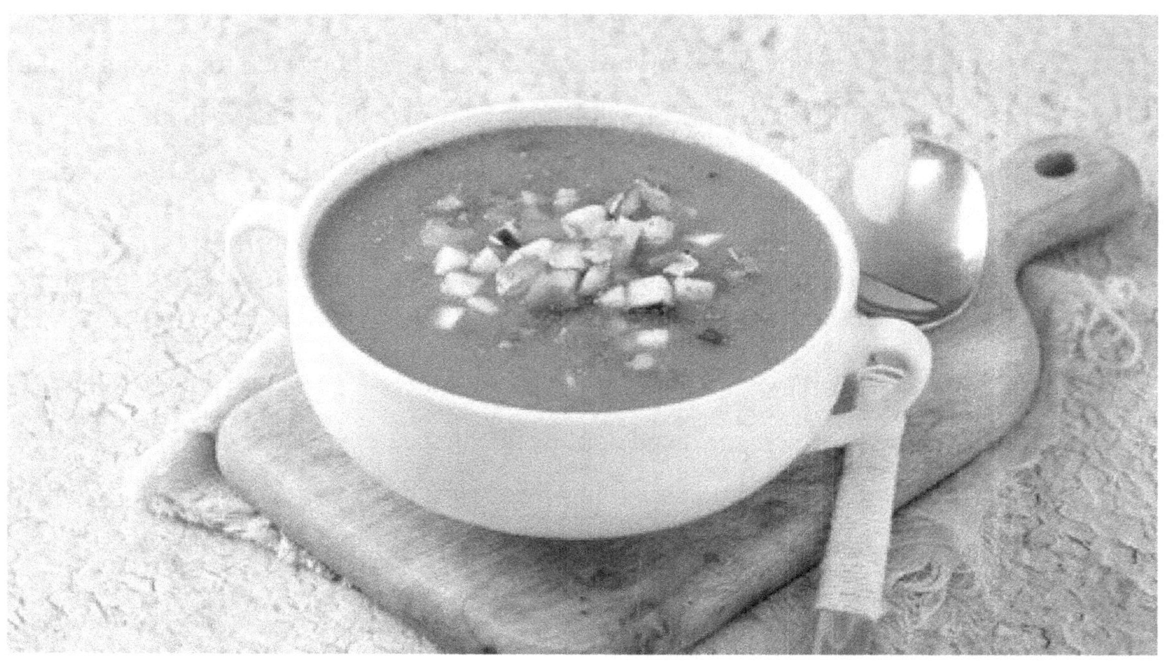

If you have ever wondered how a tomato would taste in a smoothie, here is how to find out!!

Preparation Time: 04 Minutes

Cook Time: Nil

Serve: 1

List of Ingredients:

- 1 handful of ice
- 1 chopped English cucumber
- 1 chopped carrot
- 1 handful of chopped rib celery
- 2 tbsp of water
- 1 pinch of ground cumin
- 1 tbsp of lemon juice
- 1 chopped kale leaf
- 4 tbsp of Greek yogurt
- 1 cup of diced tomatoes

AAAAAAAAAAAAAAAAAAAAAA

Methods:

A. In your smoothie maker or blender, combine the ice, chopped English cucumber, carrot, rib celery, water, ground cumin, and lemon juice.

B. Add the chopped kale leaves, Greek yogurt, and diced tomatoes to the mixture.

C. Blitz all the ingredients in the smoothie maker for about 3 minutes until you achieve a smooth and creamy consistency.

D. Serve the Tomato Kale Gazpacho immediately and enjoy this refreshing and healthy chilled soup.

Cooking Notes:

A. Gazpacho is a cold Spanish soup typically made with raw vegetables. This recipe takes a twist by incorporating kale, which adds extra nutrients and a vibrant green color to the traditional tomato gazpacho.

B. If you prefer a thinner consistency, you can add more water or vegetable broth to the mixture. Adjust the amount according to your desired thickness.

C. For extra creaminess and a tangy flavor, you can use full-fat Greek yogurt. However, if you want a lighter version, opt for low-fat Greek yogurt or substitute it with a plant-based yogurt.

D. Gazpacho is best served chilled. If you want to serve it immediately after blending, ensure that all the vegetables and yogurt are already well-chilled before starting the preparation. Alternatively, you can refrigerate the gazpacho for at least an hour before serving to enhance the flavors and allow it to reach the desired cold temperature.

E. This Tomato Kale Gazpacho can be served as a refreshing appetizer, a light lunch, or a healthy snack during hot weather.

F. Feel free to adjust the seasoning according to your taste preferences. You can add more lemon juice, cumin, or any other herbs and spices you like to enhance the flavor profile.

G. This gazpacho is highly customizable. You can add other ingredients like red bell peppers, garlic, red onions, or avocado to create different variations.

13. BBQ Prawns, Avocado and Kale

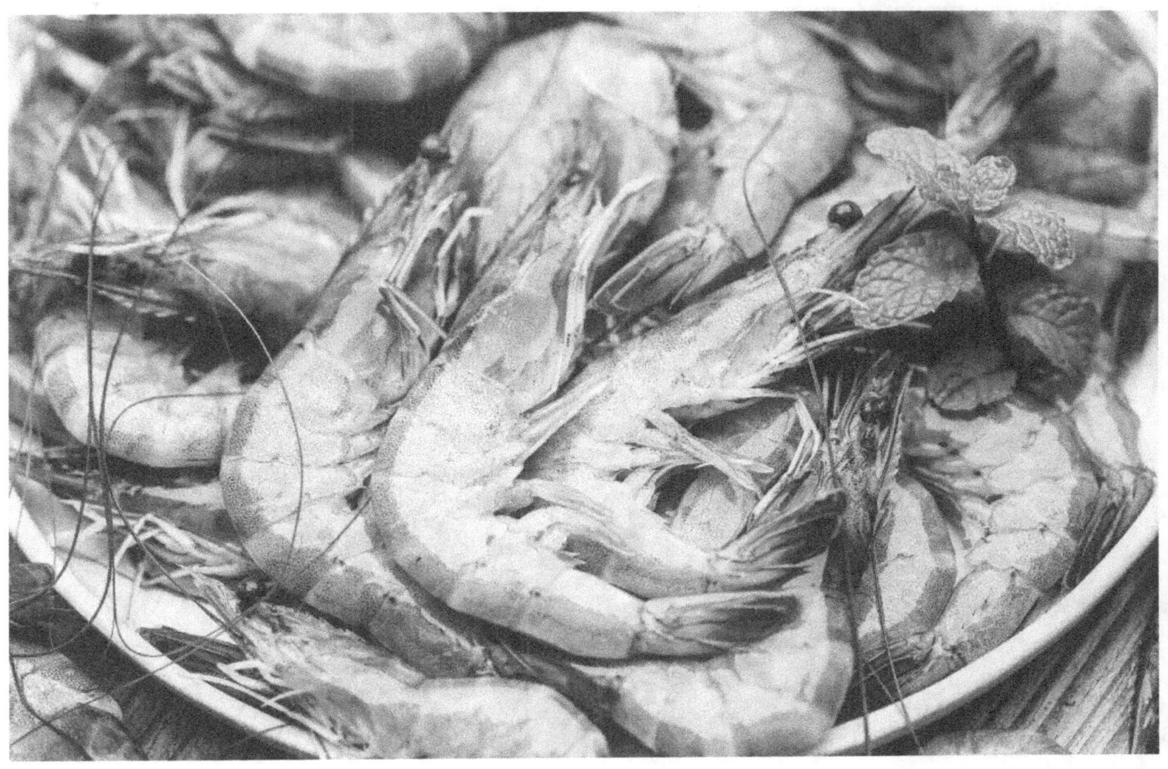

This prawn dish will give you a run for your money!

Preparation Time: 15 Minutes

Cook Time: 1 Hour

Serve: 2

List of Ingredients:

- 2 chopped long chilies (red and deseeded)
- 8 large prawns (green)
- 250g of kale
- 2 handfuls of chopped parsley leaves
- 100 ml of olive oil
- 2 tbsp of lemon juice
- 2 tbsp of grated lemon zest
- 1 minced garlic clove

AAAAAAAAAAAAAAAAAAAAAAAA

Methods:

A. Preheat the oven to 375 degrees F (190 degrees C).

B. In an ovenproof pan, mix together olive oil, black pepper, chili, and garlic. Cover the pan with foil and roast the mixture in the preheated oven for about 45 minutes until the flavors are well blended and aromatic.

C. After roasting, transfer the mixture to a blender and blend for about 3 minutes until you achieve a smooth and flavorful sauce.

D. Preheat the grill to 400 degrees F (200 degrees C).

E. Prepare the prawns by cutting them in the butterfly form, as shown in the image above. Remove the vein for a clean presentation.

F. In a bowl, combine the kale leaves with half of the roasted mixture and mix well to coat the kale with the flavorful sauce.

G. In another bowl, mix parsley with the remaining portion of the roasted mixture.

H. Rub the prawns with the parsley mixture to coat them thoroughly.

I. Grill the prawns on both sides for approximately 6 minutes until they are fully cooked and have nice grill marks.

J. Transfer the grilled prawns to a plate and garnish them with lemon juice and zest for a refreshing zing.

K. Proceed to grill the kale leaves for about 2 minutes until they are slightly charred and tender.

L. To serve, create a bed of avocado puree on the plate and arrange the grilled prawns on top. Add the grilled kale leaves as a side or garnish.

Cooking Notes:

A. The oven roasting step helps to develop the flavors of the oil, pepper, chili, and garlic. It also allows the ingredients to infuse, resulting in a more robust sauce for the dish.

B. Adjust the roasting time based on the size and thickness of the garlic cloves and chili to avoid overcooking or burning them.

C. When grilling the prawns, it's essential to keep a close eye on them as they cook quickly. Overcooking prawns can lead to a rubbery texture.

D. To butterfly the prawns, use a sharp knife to make a shallow cut along the back of the prawn, cutting through the shell and flesh. Carefully remove the vein using the tip of the knife or a toothpick.

E. You can create the avocado puree by blending ripe avocados with a little lemon juice, salt, and pepper until smooth and creamy. Adjust the seasoning to your taste preference.

F. If you prefer a spicier or milder flavor, you can adjust the amount of chili used in the roasted mixture or omit it altogether.

G. The dish can be served with a side of rice, quinoa, or crusty bread to make it a more substantial meal.

H. For added freshness, you can garnish the dish with chopped fresh herbs like cilantro or basil before serving.

14. Gnocchi and Miso Butter Prawns

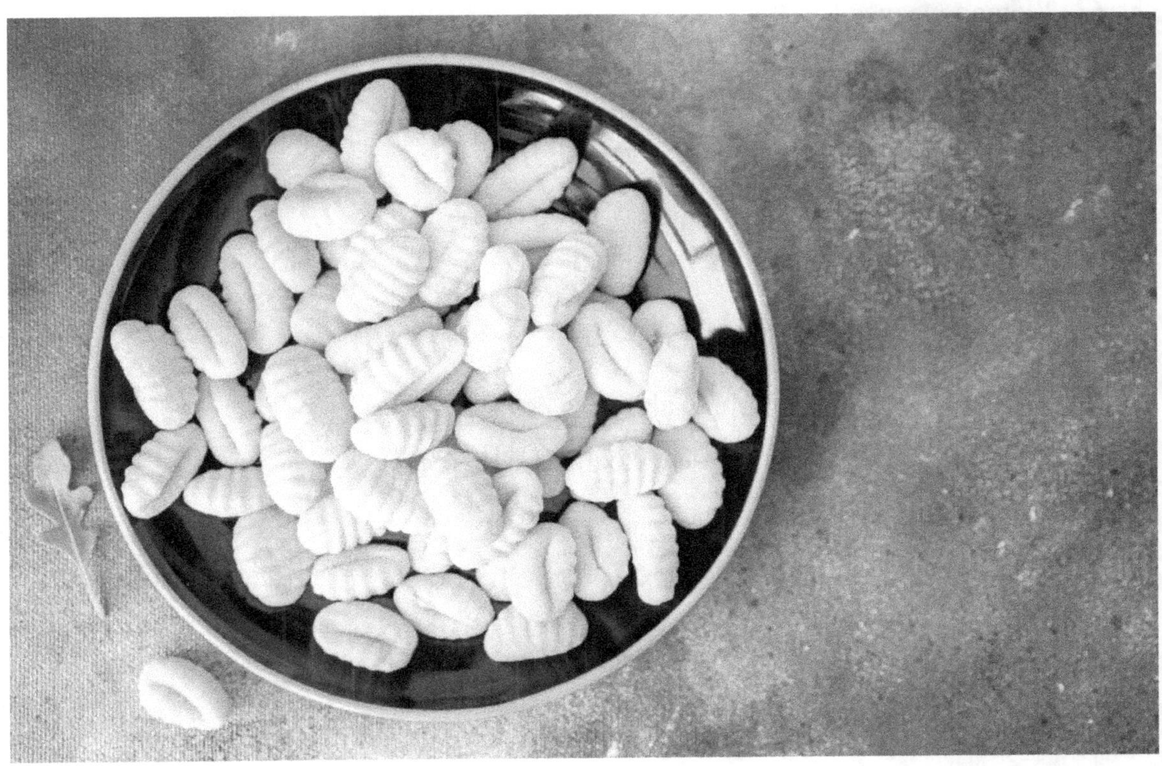

This Asian delicacy brings prawns to you in another buttery and tantalizing dimension!!

Preparation Time: 10 Minutes

Cook Time: 25 Minutes

Serve: 8

List of Ingredients:

- 4 tbsp of mirin
- 2 lemon wedges
- 500g of flour
- 4 tbsp of rice vinegar
- 4 tbsp of Miso paste (white)
- 2 tbsp of canola oil
- 4 tbsp of sesame seeds
- 2 eggs
- 1 handful of chopped purple kale
- 2kg of peeled, cooked, and deveined prawns (greens)
- 1 tbsp of lemon juice
- 200g of melted butter

AAAAAAAAAAAAAAAAAAAAAA

Methods:

A. In a pan, combine Mirin, vinegar, and Miso. Cook and stir the mixture for 3 minutes. Then, add 150g of butter and stir until melted. Finally, add lemon juice to the mixture and set it aside.

B. In a bowl, mix sesame seeds, oil, and kale well. Pour this mixture into a baking tray and bake it for 35 minutes.

C. In another bowl, combine flour and eggs to make a dough. Scoop the dough and flatten it on a floured surface. Cut it into pieces and boil them in a pan of water for about 4 minutes or until they rise to the surface. In a separate saucepan, fry the boiled gnocchi in the remaining butter until all sides are cooked. Serve the gnocchi with the Miso mixture and prawns.

Cooking Notes:

A. Mirin is a Japanese sweet rice wine that adds a subtle sweetness to the Miso butter sauce. If you don't have Mirin, you can use a mixture of rice wine vinegar and sugar as a substitute.

B. When cooking the Miso mixture, make sure to stir continuously to prevent any lumps and to evenly distribute the ingredients.

C. You can adjust the amount of Miso to suit your taste preferences. Miso has a strong umami flavor, so you can add more or less depending on how intense you want the sauce to be.

D. The baking time for the kale in the oven may vary depending on the thickness of the leaves. Check on it occasionally to avoid overcooking and ensure it becomes crispy but not burnt.

E. When making the gnocchi dough, be careful not to over-mix it, as it can make the gnocchi dense and chewy instead of light and fluffy.

F. When cutting the gnocchi into pieces, dust the knife with flour to prevent the dough from sticking to the blade.

G. To cook the gnocchi, you can drop them in boiling water and wait until they rise to the surface. This indicates that they are fully cooked. However, cooking times may vary slightly depending on the size and thickness of the gnocchi.

H. For the prawns, you can marinate them with some olive oil, garlic, salt, and pepper before cooking to enhance their flavor. Sauté the prawns in a hot pan until they are pink and cooked through.

I. To serve, arrange the cooked gnocchi on a plate, drizzle the Miso butter sauce over them, and place the prawns on top for a delicious and visually appealing dish. Garnish with some chopped green onions or sesame seeds for added flavor and presentation.

15. Zucchini and Caprese Chicken

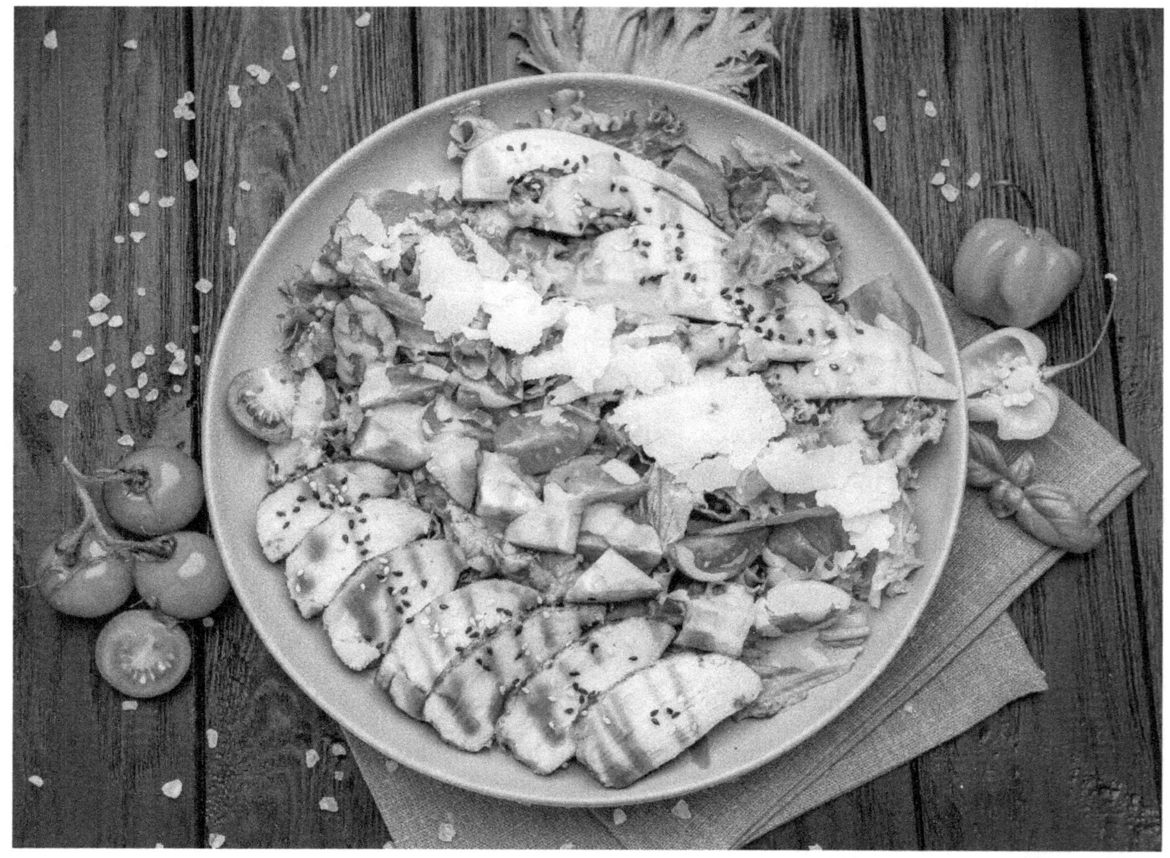

This Ukrainian and Italian combo delicacy is a masterpiece!!

Preparation Time: 10 Minutes

Cook Time: 15 Minutes

Serve: 2

List of Ingredients:

- 1 lb. of cubed boneless chicken breasts (skinless)
- 2 oz of tomato paste
- 4 oz of sliced mozzarella cheese.
- 1 tsp of salt
- 1 lb. of sliced tomatoes
- 1 tbsp of pepper
- 1 handful of sliced basil
- 1 tbsp of balsamic vinegar
- 4 minced garlic cloves
- 1 lb. of cubed zucchini
- 1 pinch of dried oregano
- 1 tbsp of oil

AAAAAAAAAAAAAAAAAAAAAA

Methods:

A. In a pan with oil, sauté the pepper and chicken together, seasoning with a pinch of salt. Cook for about 4 minutes until the chicken is browned and cooked through.

B. Push the chicken to one side of the pan and add more oil to the empty area. Sauté the garlic in the oil for about 1 minute until fragrant.

C. Add vinegar, tomatoes, oregano, tomato paste, basil, and the remaining salt to the pan. Stir everything together and cook for about 3 minutes to let the flavors meld.

D. Toss in the zucchini and mix everything in the pan thoroughly.

E. Place slices of cheese on top of the mixture and let it simmer for about 4 minutes until the cheese is melted and gooey.

F. Serve the delicious Zucchini and Caprese Chicken and enjoy this flavorful and satisfying dish.

Cooking Notes:

A. When sautéing the chicken, make sure the pan is hot, and the chicken pieces are evenly spaced to ensure they cook properly and develop a nice sear. Overcrowding the pan can lead to steaming and hinder browning.

B. Use boneless, skinless chicken breasts or thighs for this recipe. You can cut the chicken into bite-sized pieces for quicker and more even cooking.

C. If the pan becomes too dry during sautéing, you can add a little more oil or a splash of chicken broth to prevent the ingredients from sticking and burning.

D. When adding the garlic to the pan, be careful not to burn it, as burnt garlic can taste bitter and spoil the dish. Cook it just until fragrant.

E. The vinegar, tomatoes, tomato paste, and oregano contribute to the delicious sauce for the dish. You can adjust the amount of tomato paste and vinegar to your taste preference. If you prefer a thicker sauce, you can add more tomato paste, and if you like it tangier, you can add more vinegar.

F. For the cheese, you can use fresh mozzarella or any other melting cheese of your choice. Slicing or tearing the cheese into pieces ensures even distribution over the pan.

G. While simmering the dish with the cheese on top, you can cover the pan with a lid to help the cheese melt faster and more evenly.

H. You can garnish the dish with some fresh basil leaves or a sprinkle of grated Parmesan cheese before serving to enhance the flavors and add a visual appeal.

I. Zucchini and Caprese Chicken can be served as is or over cooked pasta, rice, or quinoa for a more substantial meal.

16. Shrimp Stir Fry

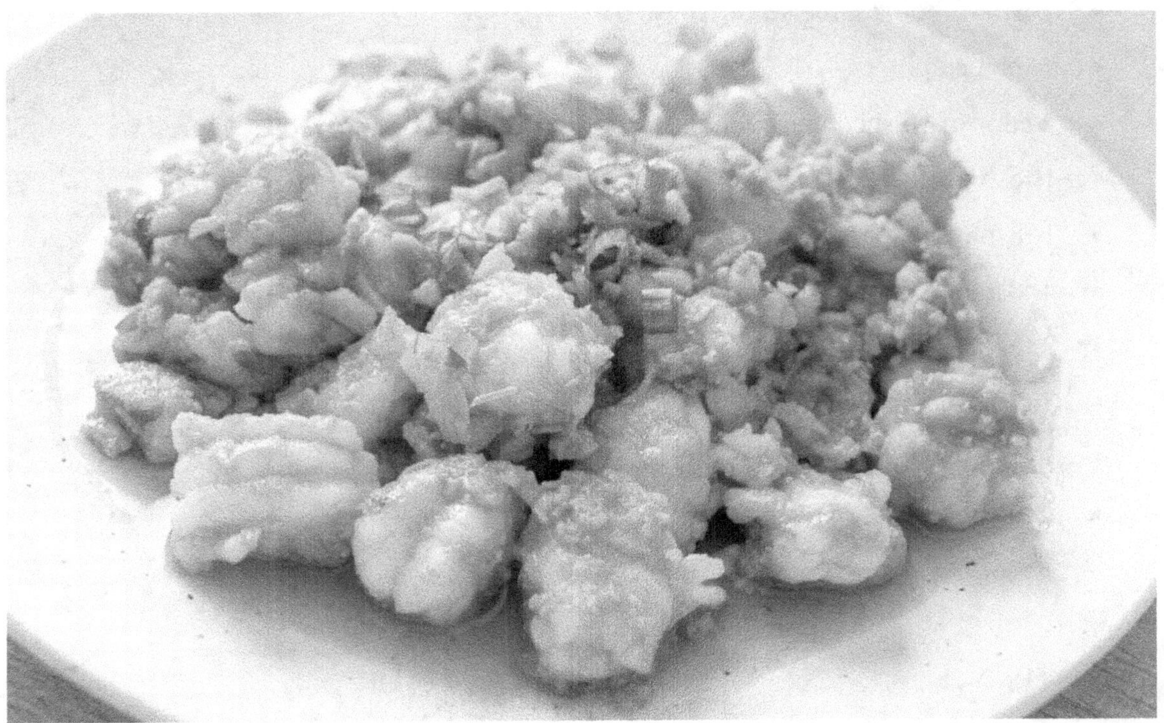

Let's try this previous recipe with shrimp!! Something colorful and delicious for shrimp lovers!

Preparation Time: 05 Minutes

Cook Time: 10 Minutes

Serve: 2

List of Ingredients:

- 2 cups of chopped desired vegetables
- 1 handful of sesame seeds (toasted)
- 1 minced ginger
- 2 cups of washed and peeled shrimp (deveined)
- 1 tbsp of rice vinegar
- 1 tbsp of pepper
- 4 tbsp of soy sauce
- 2 tbsp of sesame oil
- 2 minced garlic cloves
- 1 tbsp of sugar (brown)
- 1 tbsp of salt

AAAAAAAAAAAAAAAAAAAAAA

Methods:

A. In a skillet, sauté the ginger and garlic in oil for about 2 minutes until they become fragrant.
B. Add the shrimps to the skillet and cook them for approximately 6 minutes until they turn pink and are fully cooked.
C. Stir in the vegetables, vinegar, and sauce, and cook everything together for about 3 minutes to allow the flavors to meld.
D. Season the stir-fry with sugar, pepper, and salt, and toss all the ingredients well to ensure they are evenly coated with the flavorful sauce.
E. Serve the delicious Shrimp Stir Fry and garnish it with sesame seeds for added texture and nutty flavor.

Cooking Notes:

A. When sautéing the ginger and garlic, be careful not to burn them, as burnt garlic can taste bitter and spoil the dish. Cook them just until fragrant and lightly golden.

B. For the shrimps, you can use fresh or frozen ones. If using frozen shrimps, make sure to thaw them thoroughly before cooking. Pat the shrimps dry with paper towels to remove excess moisture, which helps them sear better and prevents them from becoming soggy.

C. Use a mix of colorful vegetables like bell peppers, snap peas, carrots, and broccoli for a vibrant and nutritious stir-fry. Cut the vegetables into similar-sized pieces for even cooking.

D. The sauce can be a combination of soy sauce, oyster sauce, and a splash of sesame oil. Adjust the amount of sauce to your taste preference, and you can also add other seasonings like garlic chili sauce or honey for additional depth of flavor.

E. To make the sauce thicker and glossy, you can add a cornstarch slurry (cornstarch mixed with water) during the last minute of cooking. Stir the slurry into the pan and cook until the sauce thickens.

F. Taste and adjust the seasoning according to your preference. You can add more sugar for sweetness, more pepper for spiciness, or more salt for overall seasoning.

G. Serve the Shrimp Stir Fry over steamed rice or noodles for a complete and satisfying meal. You can also garnish it with sliced green onions or fresh cilantro for extra freshness and visual appeal.

H. Customize the stir-fry with your favorite vegetables and spices to suit your taste. Stir-fries are versatile dishes that can easily be adapted to include various ingredients and flavors.

17. Happy Green Monster

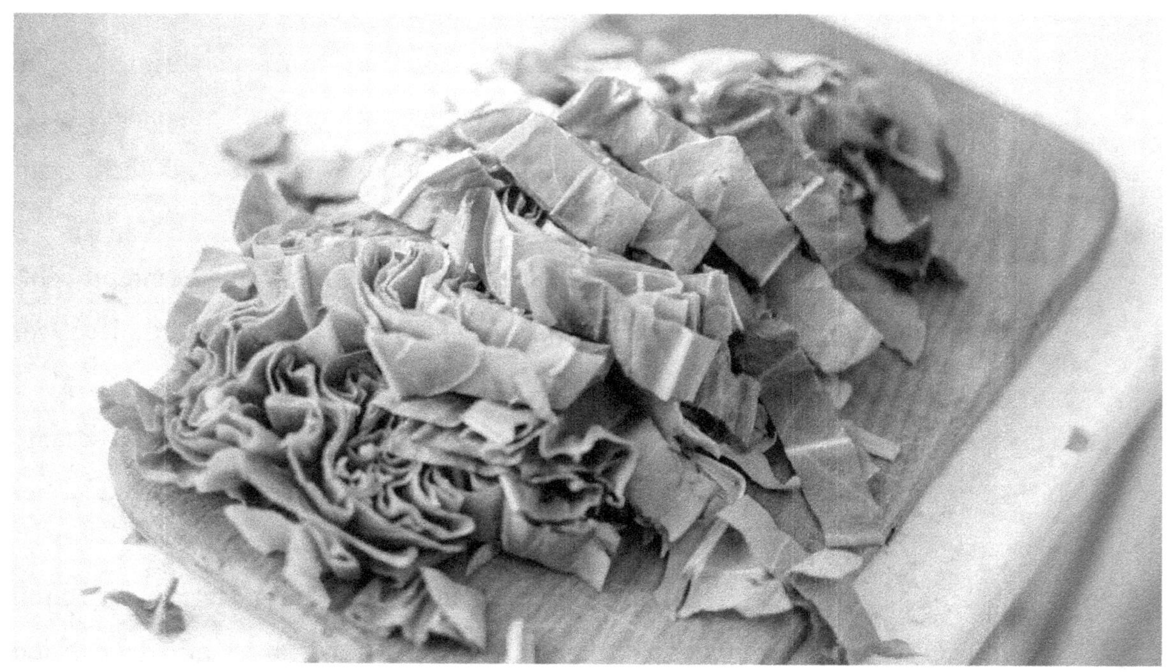

Monster???!!!

Preparation Time: 04 Minutes

Cook Time: Nil

Serve: 1

List of Ingredients:

- 8 tbsp of coconut water
- 1 handful of chopped kale
- 1 handful of chopped spinach
- 3 tbsp of coconut milk
- 1 cored and peeled pear (chopped)
- 3 tbsp of lemon juice
- 1 tsp of agave syrup

AAAAAAAAAAAAAAAAAAAAAA

Methods:

A. In your blender, add 8 tbsp of coconut water, a handful of chopped kale, a handful of chopped spinach, 3 tbsp of coconut milk, and a cored and peeled pear (chopped).
B. Pour in 3 tbsp of lemon juice and add 1 tsp of agave syrup for sweetness.
C. Blend all the ingredients together until you get a smooth and creamy texture.
D. Stir the mixture to ensure it is well combined, then serve and enjoy your Happy Green Monster smoothie!

Cooking Notes:

A. You can customize this Happy Green Monster smoothie by adding other green ingredients like cucumber, celery, or avocado for added nutrition and flavor.
B. If you prefer a thicker consistency, you can add ice cubes or frozen fruits to the blender before blending.
C. Feel free to adjust the sweetness level by adding more or less agave syrup, honey, or any other sweetener of your choice.

D. For an extra boost of nutrients, you can add superfood ingredients like chia seeds, flaxseeds, or protein powder to the blender.

E. To make it a complete meal, you can add a scoop of your favorite protein powder or nut butter to increase the protein content.

F. Greens Variety: Feel free to experiment with different leafy greens in this smoothie. Aside from kale and spinach, you can try adding arugula, Swiss chard, or even beet greens for a unique flavor and additional nutrients.

G. Using Frozen Fruits: If you want a colder and thicker smoothie without diluting the flavor with ice, you can use frozen fruits like frozen pineapple, frozen mango, or frozen banana. Frozen fruits not only add creaminess but also retain more nutrients.

H. Coconut Water Alternatives: If you don't have coconut water on hand, you can substitute it with regular water or almond milk for a slightly nutty taste. Alternatively, use fresh coconut water if you have access to young coconuts.

I. Ripe Pear: For the best taste and sweetness, use a ripe and juicy pear. If your pear is not very ripe, you can add a little more agave syrup or honey to compensate for the lack of natural sweetness.

J. Agave Syrup Substitute: If you prefer to avoid agave syrup, you can use other natural sweeteners like maple syrup, date syrup, or stevia. Adjust the amount based on your desired level of sweetness.

K. Prepping Ahead: To save time in the morning, you can pre-portion and freeze the greens and chopped pear in individual bags or containers. This way, you can quickly grab the ingredients and blend them without any fuss.

L. Optional Boosters: For added nutrition, consider incorporating adaptogens like spirulina, matcha powder, or wheatgrass into the smoothie. These ingredients can provide an extra health boost.

M. Storage: If you have leftover smoothie, store it in an airtight container in the refrigerator. Give it a good shake or stir before drinking, as the ingredients may naturally separate over time.

N. Hydration: The coconut water in this smoothie helps keep you hydrated, making it an excellent choice for staying refreshed during hot weather or after a workout.

O. Sip Slowly: Enjoy this Happy Green Monster smoothie slowly to savor its vibrant flavors and allow your body to absorb all the nutrients. Drinking it mindfully can also help with digestion and satiety.

P. The Happy Green Monster smoothie is a versatile and nutrient-rich drink that can be tailored to suit your taste and health preferences. With its combination of greens, fruits, and coconut goodness, it's a delightful way to kickstart your day or recharge your energy levels. Enjoy this vibrant and nourishing green smoothie as a part of your daily wellness routine!

18. Oats and Flax Smoothie

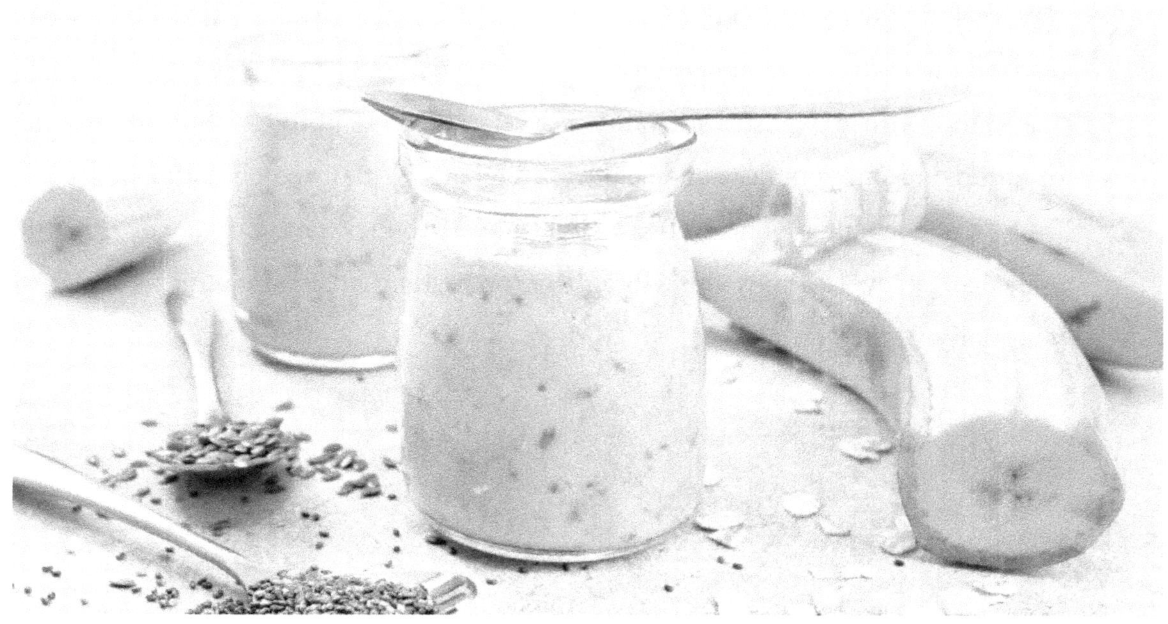

This smoothie contains all that your sweet tooth craves in a smoothie!!

Preparation Time: 04 Minutes

Cook Time: Nil

Serve: 1

List of Ingredients:

- 1 chopped banana
- 1 tbsp of flax seed
- 1 handful of whole grain granola
- 4 tbsp of milk
- 2 handfuls of raw rolled oats
- 1 handful of spinach

AAAAAAAAAAAAAAAAAAAAAAA

Methods:

A. In a blender, combine the milk, banana, and spinach.

B. Blend the ingredients until smooth and creamy, creating a nutritious and delicious base for the Oats and Flax Smoothie.

C. Pour the smoothie into a glass and garnish it with flax seeds, oats, and granola for added texture and health benefits.

D. Now, your Oats and Flax Smoothie is ready to be enjoyed! Sip on this wholesome and filling smoothie, packed with fiber, vitamins, and minerals.

Cooking Notes:

A. The milk used in the recipe can be any type of milk you prefer, such as almond milk, soy milk, or cow's milk. Choose the one that suits your taste and dietary needs.

B. For the banana, using a ripe and sweet banana will add natural sweetness to the smoothie, eliminating the need for additional sweeteners. If you like a stronger banana flavor, you can add more banana slices to the blender.

C. Spinach is a great addition to the smoothie as it provides essential nutrients like iron, vitamin C, and fiber. You can use fresh or frozen spinach, depending on what you have available.

D. To enhance the nutritional content, consider adding other ingredients to the blender, such as chia seeds, hemp seeds, or a scoop of protein powder. These additions will increase the smoothie's protein content and keep you feeling fuller for longer.

E. When garnishing with flax seeds, oats, and granola, you can use them in varying amounts according to your preference. These toppings not only add a delightful crunch but also contribute to the overall nutritional value of the smoothie.

F. If you like a colder and creamier texture, you can add some ice cubes to the blender before blending the ingredients. This will create a refreshing and frosty smoothie.

G. Feel free to customize the smoothie by adding other fruits like berries, mango, or pineapple for different flavors and nutrients.

H. Soaking Oats: If you prefer a smoother texture and easier digestion, you can soak the oats in the milk for 10-15 minutes before blending. Soaking softens the oats and makes them creamier in the smoothie.

I. Sweeteners: While the ripe banana provides natural sweetness, you can add a touch of honey, maple syrup, or a few dates to the blender if you desire a sweeter smoothie.

J. Nut Butters: For a nutty flavor and added creaminess, consider blending in a tablespoon of almond butter, peanut butter, or cashew butter. This addition also boosts the smoothie's protein content.

K. Flaxseed Benefits: Flaxseeds are rich in omega-3 fatty acids, fiber, and lignans. To maximize their nutritional benefits, consider grinding the flax seeds before adding them to the blender. Ground flaxseeds are easier to digest and allow better nutrient absorption.

L. Make-Ahead: If you're short on time in the morning, you can prepare the ingredients for the smoothie the night before. Place the milk, banana, and spinach in a sealed container and store it in the refrigerator. In the morning, simply blend the prepped ingredients with the additional toppings.

M. Greens Variety: While spinach is an excellent choice for this smoothie, you can experiment with other leafy greens like kale, Swiss chard, or collard greens for different flavors and nutrients.

N. Protein Options: To increase the protein content of the smoothie, you can add a scoop of your favorite protein powder, such as whey protein, pea protein, or plant-based protein.

O. Preparing Frozen Ingredients: If you prefer a colder and thicker smoothie, you can freeze the banana and spinach in advance. Simply slice the banana and store it in a sealed bag in the freezer. For the spinach, blanch it quickly in boiling water, then drain and freeze it in portions.

P. Chilled Glass: For an extra refreshing experience, chill the glass in the refrigerator or freezer before pouring the smoothie into it.

Q. Experiment with Spices: If you enjoy spices, consider adding a pinch of ground cinnamon, nutmeg, or ginger to the blender. These spices not only add depth to the flavor but also provide additional health benefits.

R. The Oats and Flax Smoothie is a versatile and nutrient-packed way to start your day or recharge after a workout. With its customizable ingredients and easy preparation, it's a delicious and wholesome addition to your smoothie repertoire. Enjoy this nourishing treat and get creative with your own favorite toppings and variations!

19. Spinach and Orange Smoothie

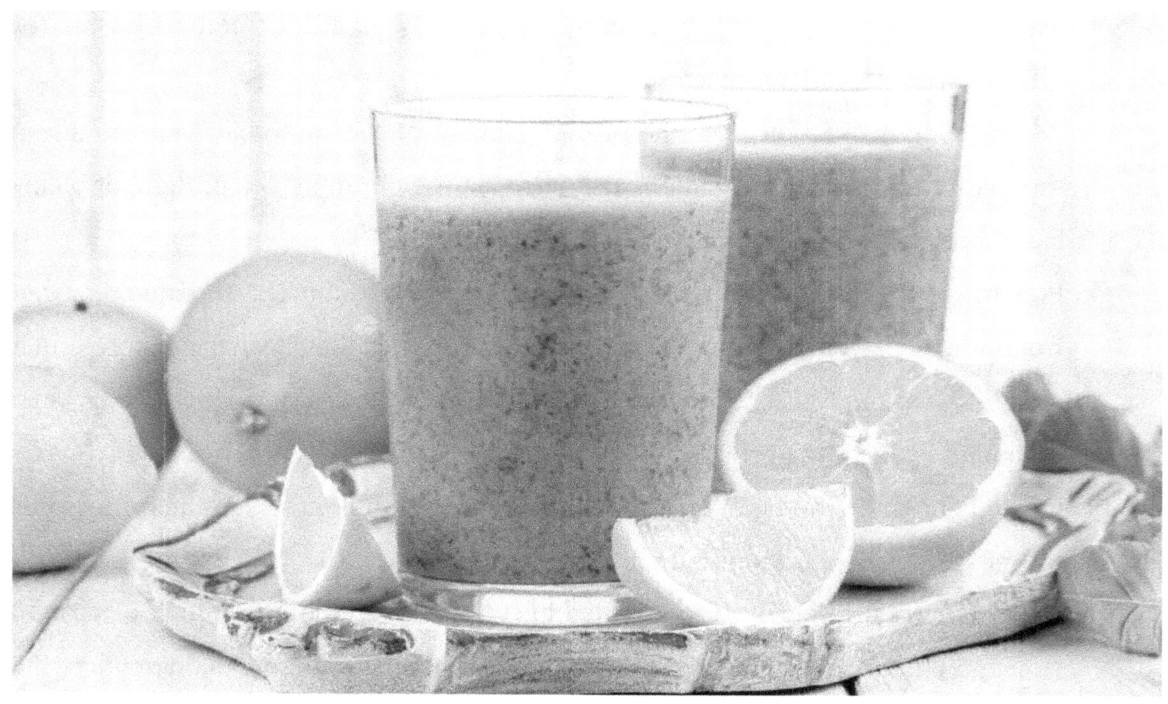

This creamy and citrusy smoothie is the perfect drink for you to start up your day!!!!

Preparation Time: 03 Minutes

Cook Time: Nil

Serve: 1

List of Ingredients:

- 1 chopped banana
- 1 orange (peeled)
- 6 tbsp of coconut water
- 1 handful of chopped spinach
- 1 cup of ice

AAAAAAAAAAAAAAAAAAAAAA

Methods:

A. In a blender, combine the chopped banana, peeled orange, chopped spinach, and coconut water. The banana adds natural sweetness, the orange provides a refreshing citrus flavor, and the coconut water adds a hint of tropical taste.

B. Add a cup of ice to the blender to create a chilled and refreshing smoothie with a pleasant texture.

C. Blend all the ingredients together until smooth and creamy. This should take about 1-2 minutes, depending on the power of your blender.

D. Pour the Spinach and Orange Smoothie into glasses and serve immediately. This delightful and nutritious drink is ready to be enjoyed as a quick and healthy snack or a refreshing breakfast option.

Cooking Notes:

A. For the coconut water, you can use store-bought coconut water or freshly extracted coconut water from a young coconut. Coconut water is not only a great source of hydration but also adds a subtle tropical flavor to the smoothie.

B. When using fresh oranges, make sure to peel them to remove the bitter pith and retain only the juicy segments. This will ensure a sweeter and more pleasant taste in the smoothie.

C. The ice is added to the blender to create a chilled and slushy consistency. However, if you prefer a thicker smoothie, you can skip the ice and use frozen banana or add more chopped spinach to achieve the desired texture.

D. To enhance the nutritional content of the smoothie, consider adding additional ingredients like chia seeds, flaxseeds, or a scoop of protein powder. These additions will boost the smoothie's fiber and protein content, making it even more satisfying and nutritious.

E. Spinach is rich in vitamins, minerals, and antioxidants. It is a fantastic addition to any smoothie as it adds a vibrant green color without overpowering the taste.

F. The sweetness of the smoothie comes from the natural sugars present in the banana and orange. If you prefer a sweeter smoothie, you can add a drizzle of honey, maple syrup, or any other sweetener of your choice.

G. Greens Variation: While spinach is the star of this smoothie, you can also experiment with other greens like kale, Swiss chard, or arugula. Each green brings its unique flavor and nutritional benefits to the smoothie.

H. Orange Zest: For a burst of citrus aroma and flavor, consider adding a little bit of orange zest to the blender. The zest contains essential oils that can enhance the overall taste of the smoothie.

I. Nut Butter Boost: To add creaminess and a nutty flavor to the smoothie, you can blend in a tablespoon of almond butter, peanut butter, or cashew butter. This addition also adds healthy fats and protein to make the smoothie more satisfying.

J. Herbal Twist: Add a few fresh mint leaves or a sprig of basil to the blender for a refreshing herbal twist. The combination of mint or basil with the orange and spinach creates a delightful and aromatic flavor profile.

K. Preparing Frozen Fruit: If you want to use frozen fruits instead of ice for a thicker smoothie, make sure to chop and freeze the banana and orange segments in advance. Freezing the fruits helps to maintain their freshness and prevents them from diluting the smoothie's flavor.

L. Non-Dairy Milk: If you prefer a creamier consistency, you can replace the coconut water with your favorite non-dairy milk, such as almond milk, oat milk, or soy milk.

M. Serving in Bowls: Transform this smoothie into a nutritious and beautiful smoothie bowl by pouring it into a bowl and adding toppings like sliced fruits, granola, chia seeds, or coconut flakes.

N. Hydration Tips: If you plan to enjoy this smoothie after a workout or during a hot day, consider adding a pinch of salt to the blender. The salt helps replenish electrolytes lost through sweating.

O. Adjusting Texture: If the smoothie turns out too thick, you can add more coconut water or regular water to achieve the desired consistency.

P. Make-Ahead: While this smoothie is best consumed immediately, you can prepare the ingredients in advance and store them in separate containers. When ready to enjoy, simply add the ingredients to the blender and blend until smooth.

Q. The Spinach and Orange Smoothie is a wonderful way to incorporate leafy greens and fruits into your diet while enjoying a refreshing and delicious beverage. Whether you're a smoothie enthusiast or a beginner, this recipe is a great addition to your repertoire of healthy and easy-to-make drinks. Sip, savor, and nourish your body with this vibrant green goodness!

20. Skillet Enchiladas

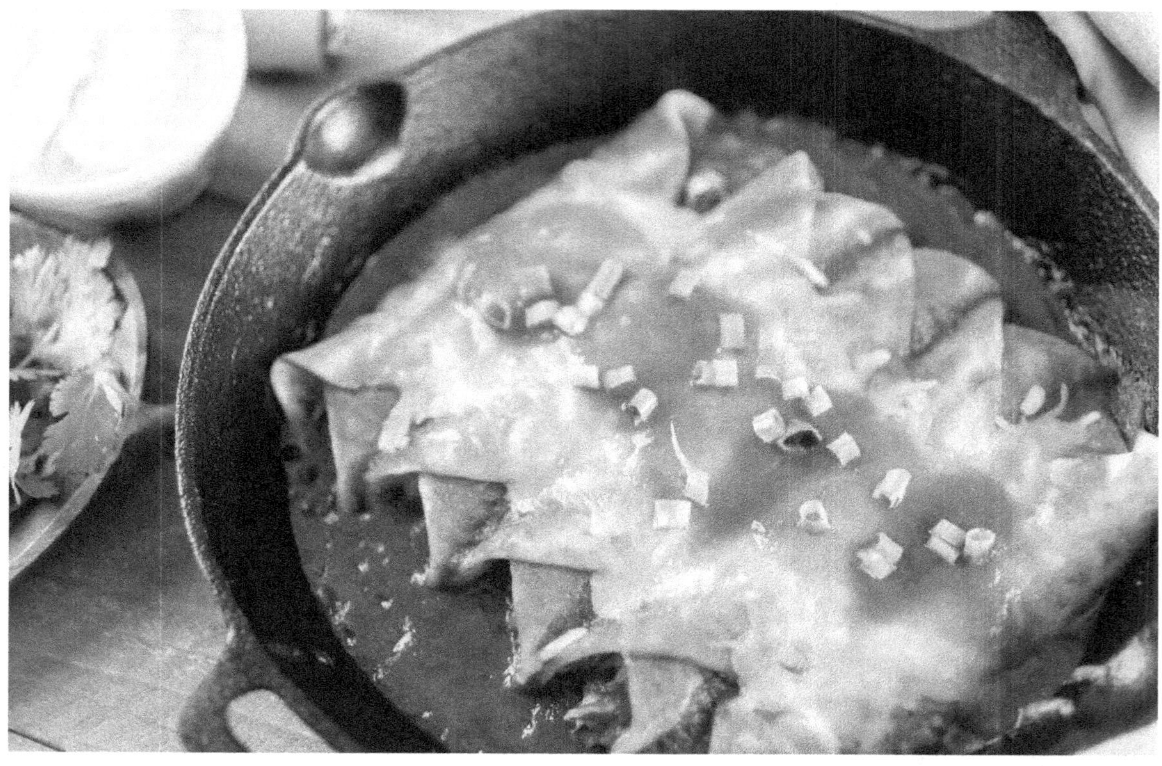

Do you need something light but healthy and tantalizing for a quick dinner? Here is it!!

Preparation Time: 05 Minutes

Cook Time: 15 Minutes

Serve: 3

List of Ingredients:

- 5 wheat tortillas (in strips)
- 7 oz of drained black beans (rinsed)
- 1 chopped medium-sized onion
- 1 tbsp of cumin
- 7 oz of tomato sauce
- 1 tbsp of honey
- 3 oz of tomato paste
- 1 tbsp of pepper
- 2 minced garlic cloves
- 1 pound of lean beef (ground)
- 1 cup of corn
- 6 tbsp of broth
- 1 cup of shredded cheddar cheese
- 1 tbsp of chili powder
- 1 pinch of salt

AAAAAAAAAAAAAAAAAAAAAA

Methods:

A. In a skillet, sauté the ground beef, garlic, onion, chili, pepper, salt, and cumin. Cook the mixture for about 7 minutes until the beef is browned and the onions and garlic are fragrant.

B. Add the honey, tomato paste, enchilada sauce, water, tortillas, corn, and black beans to the skillet. Stir everything together to ensure all the ingredients are well combined.

C. Cover the skillet with a lid and let it cook for an additional 8 minutes. This allows the flavors to meld together and the tortillas to soften.

D. Once the skillet enchiladas are fully cooked, sprinkle shredded cheese on top. Cover the skillet again for a few minutes until the cheese melts and becomes gooey and delicious.

E. To serve, dish out the skillet enchiladas onto plates. Garnish each serving with a dollop of yogurt or sour cream for a creamy element and a sprinkle of chopped green onions for added freshness and color.

Cooking Notes:

A. You can use either ground beef or ground turkey for this recipe, depending on your preference or dietary restrictions. Both options work well and provide a hearty and satisfying filling for the enchiladas.

B. Adjust the amount of chili powder and cumin according to your spice preference. If you like it mild, use less chili powder or remove the seeds and membranes from the chili before adding it to the skillet.

C. The honey in the recipe adds a touch of sweetness and balances the savory flavors. You can adjust the amount of honey to suit your taste.

D. Corn and black beans add texture and flavor to the dish, but you can also customize the filling by adding other vegetables like bell peppers, zucchini, or spinach. Be creative with the filling to cater to your taste and dietary needs.

E. Enchilada sauce is typically available in stores, or you can make your own using canned or fresh tomatoes, chili, garlic, and spices. If using store-bought sauce, choose your preferred level of spiciness or try different varieties to find your favorite.

F. For the tortillas, you can use corn tortillas or flour tortillas. Corn tortillas offer a more traditional flavor and texture, while flour tortillas tend to be softer and slightly sweeter. Warm the tortillas slightly before adding them to the skillet for easier rolling and cooking.

G. Optional Garnishes: Besides yogurt or sour cream and chopped green onions, you can get creative with other garnishing options. Chopped cilantro, sliced jalapenos, diced avocado, or a squeeze of lime juice can add different layers of flavors and textures to the dish.

H. Preparing the Tortillas: To prevent the tortillas from tearing or becoming soggy, you can lightly fry or heat them on a dry skillet before adding them to the enchilada mixture. This step helps to enhance their pliability and maintain their structure.

I. Enchilada Sauce Variations: If you enjoy a smokier flavor, you can use chipotle-based enchilada sauce instead of regular enchilada sauce. Chipotle sauce adds a delicious smoky kick to the dish.

J. Make-Ahead Option: This skillet enchilada recipe can be assembled ahead of time and refrigerated until you are ready to cook it. Simply cover the skillet with plastic wrap or aluminum foil and store it in the refrigerator until you're ready to cook. You may need to adjust the cooking time slightly if starting with a cold skillet.

K. Toppings for Serving: When serving the skillet enchiladas, offer a variety of toppings on the side so that everyone can customize their dish according to their taste. Salsa, guacamole, sliced jalapenos, shredded lettuce, or diced tomatoes can all be delightful additions.

L. Leftovers: Store any leftover skillet enchiladas in an airtight container in the refrigerator. To reheat, you can use the stovetop on low heat or microwave them. Add a splash of water or enchilada sauce while reheating to prevent them from drying out.

M. Tortilla Chip Topping: If you have some tortilla chips on hand, you can crush them and sprinkle them over the skillet enchiladas before serving. The chips add a delightful crunch and an extra layer of flavor to the dish.

N. Adjusting Spiciness: If you find the dish too spicy, you can temper the heat by increasing the amount of honey or adding a dollop of sour cream when serving.

O. Skillet enchiladas are a versatile and comforting dish that brings together the vibrant flavors of Mexican cuisine in a one-pan meal. With the ability to customize the filling and toppings, it's a fantastic recipe to make your own and enjoy with your loved ones. Whether you're cooking for a weeknight dinner or a gathering, these delicious and hearty enchiladas are sure to please!

21. Canja de Galinha

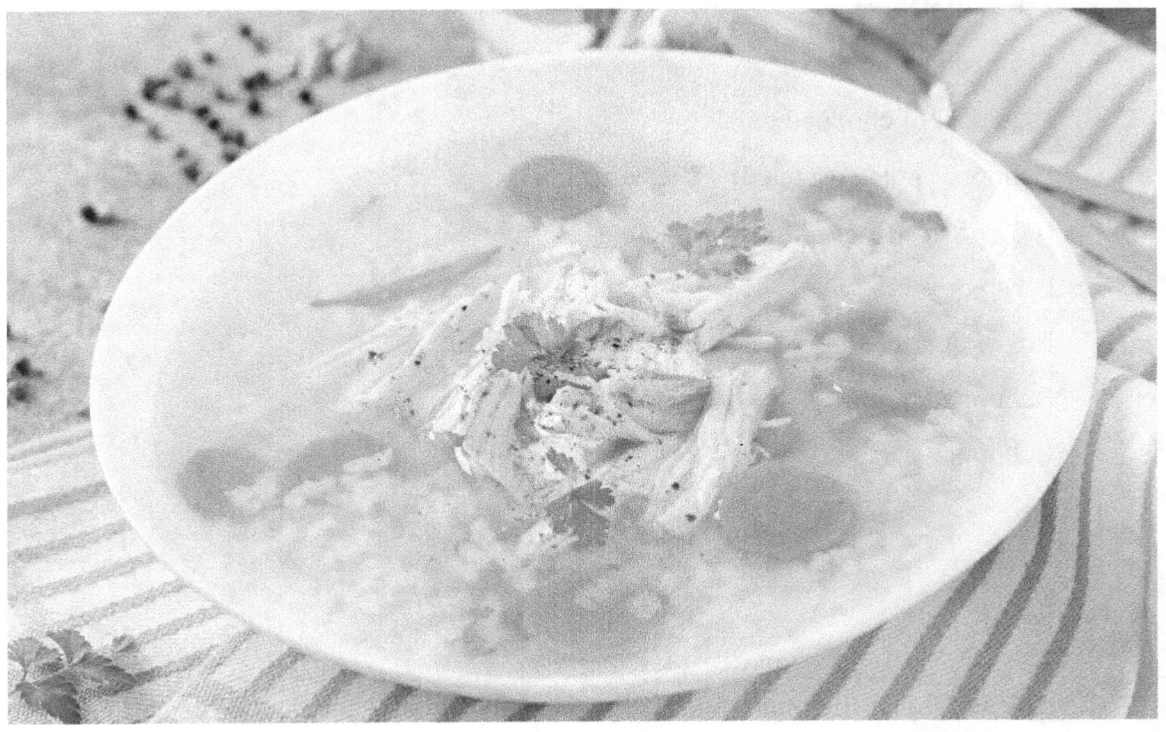

Let's pitch our tent in Brazil with this one!!!

Preparation Time: 10 Minutes

Cook Time: 25 Minutes

Serve: 2

List of Ingredients:

- 1 l of chicken stock
- 1 tbsp of pepper
- 1 minced garlic clove
- 1 handful of chopped parsley
- 1 chopper potato (peeled)
- 100g of rice (long-grain)
- 1 tbsp of oil
- 1kg of quartered skinless chicken (shredded)
- 1 chopped onion
- 1 chopped carrot

AAAAAAAAAAAAAAAAAAAAAAA

Methods:

A. In a pan, sauté the onion and garlic in oil for about 3 minutes. This step helps to release the flavors of the onion and garlic and create a fragrant base for the soup.

B. Add the stock, chicken, vegetables, pepper, rice, and salt to the pan. The stock serves as the base liquid for the soup, and the chicken, vegetables, rice, and seasonings add depth and richness to the dish.

C. Cook the mixture for about 20 minutes, or until the chicken is fully cooked and the rice and vegetables are tender. The cooking time may vary depending on the size of the chicken pieces and the type of vegetables used. Stir occasionally to ensure even cooking.

D. Once the Canja de Galinha is fully cooked, serve it in bowls and garnish with chopped parsley. The parsley adds a fresh, herbaceous flavor and a pop of color to the dish.

Cooking Notes:

A. Canja de Galinha is a traditional Portuguese chicken and rice soup that is known for its comforting and nourishing qualities. It is often served as a remedy for colds and a comforting meal for those feeling under the weather.

B. For the stock, you can use homemade chicken stock or store-bought chicken broth. If using store-bought broth, choose low-sodium or no-salt-added varieties, as the dish already contains salt.

C. When sautéing the onion and garlic, be careful not to let them brown too much, as this can impart a bitter taste to the soup. Aim for a soft, translucent texture for the onions and a light golden color for the garlic.

D. The type of vegetables used in Canja de Galinha can vary. Traditionally, carrots and peas are commonly added, but you can also include other vegetables such as celery, potatoes, or bell peppers to enhance the flavors and textures.

E. You can use bone-in chicken pieces (like chicken thighs or drumsticks) or boneless, skinless chicken breasts for this recipe. Bone-in chicken will add more flavor to the soup, while boneless chicken breasts will result in a leaner and lighter version.

F. Adjust the seasoning to your taste. If you prefer a spicier soup, you can add a pinch of crushed red pepper flakes or a dash of hot sauce. Additionally, you can add a squeeze of lemon juice for a slightly tangy flavor.

G. Canja de Galinha is a versatile soup, and you can customize it to suit your preferences. Some variations include adding cooked white beans or using quinoa instead of rice for a different twist.

H. Leftovers of Canja de Galinha can be stored in the refrigerator for a few days. The soup may thicken upon refrigeration; you can add some water or broth when reheating to bring it back to the desired consistency.

I. Preparing the Chicken: If using bone-in chicken pieces, you can brown them in the pan before sautéing the onion and garlic. This step adds extra flavor to the soup by caramelizing the chicken. Remove the browned chicken from the pan, set it aside, and proceed with sautéing the onion and garlic. Add the browned chicken back to the pan when adding the stock and vegetables.

J. Herbs and Spices: Besides parsley, you can add other herbs and spices to enhance the flavor of Canja de Galinha. Fresh thyme, bay leaves, or a small piece of cinnamon stick are traditional additions that can infuse the soup with warm and aromatic notes.

K. Chicken Skimming: While the soup is simmering, you may notice some foam or impurities rising to the surface. You can skim off this foam with a spoon to achieve a cleaner and clearer broth.

L. Chicken Broth Tips: If using store-bought chicken broth, choose a high-quality brand with natural ingredients and no artificial additives. To enhance the flavor of the broth, you can simmer it with the chicken bones and vegetable trimmings before straining it for use in the soup.

M. Vegetable Variations: Feel free to use seasonal vegetables or any vegetables you have on hand. Corn, green beans, or chopped kale can be wonderful additions to add variety and nutrition to the soup.

N. Rice Texture: The type of rice used can affect the texture of the soup. Short-grain rice will release more starch and create a creamier consistency, while long-grain rice will result in a lighter and fluffier texture.

O. Soup Consistency: If the soup is too thick for your liking, you can add more chicken broth or water to reach the desired consistency.

P. Serving Accompaniments: Canja de Galinha is often served with additional condiments like a drizzle of olive oil, a sprinkle of freshly ground black pepper, or a squeeze of lemon juice. These little touches can elevate the flavors and complement the soup beautifully.

Q. Make-Ahead: This soup can be made ahead of time and reheated before serving. When reheating, you may need to add a bit of water or broth to adjust the consistency.

R. Freezing: Canja de Galinha can be frozen in airtight containers for up to three months. Thaw in the refrigerator overnight and reheat on the stove or in the microwave.

S. Enjoy Canja de Galinha as a hearty and comforting soup that brings warmth and nourishment to your table. It's a versatile dish that can be adjusted to suit your preferences and dietary needs, making it a beloved recipe for many occasions.

22. Spag and Tomato Sauce

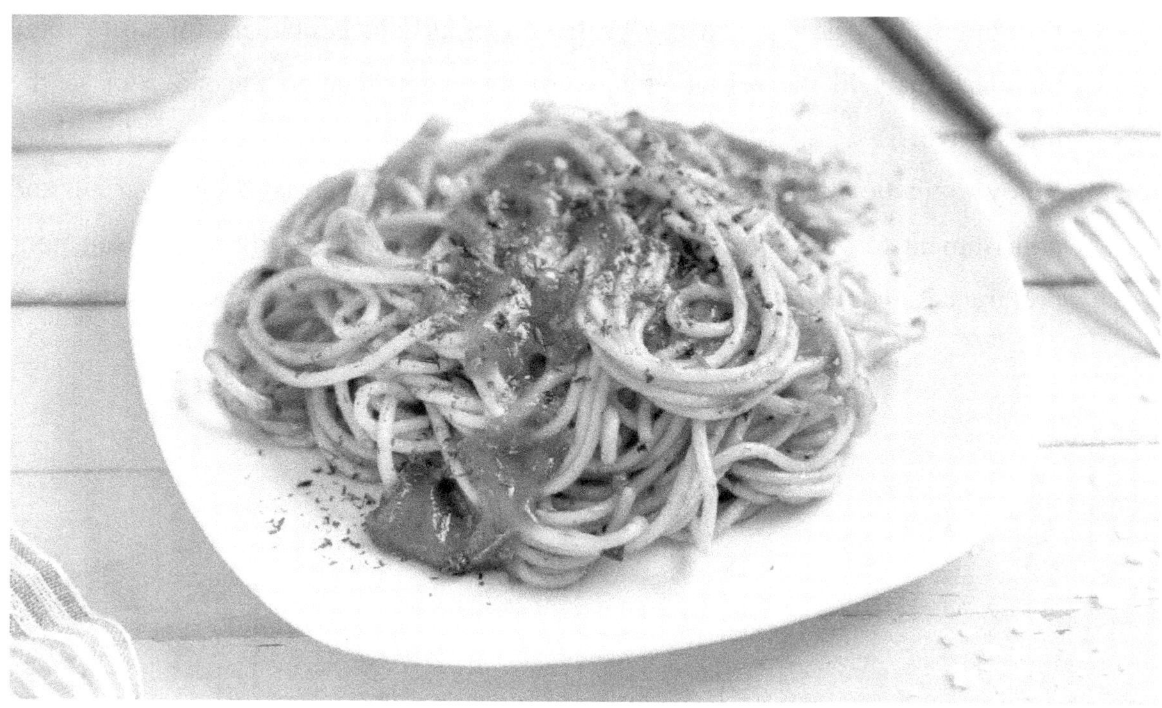

Why throw your money away in an Italian restaurant when you can simply recreate this in your kitchen?!

Preparation Time: 02 Minutes

Cook Time: 08 Minutes

Serve: 2

List of Ingredients:

- 8 oz of cooked spaghetti (drained)
- 1 tbsp of salt
- 3 minced garlic cloves
- 1 tbsp of dried oregano
- 2 tbsp of grated Parmesan cheese
- 1 tbsp of olive oil
- 1 tbsp of pepper
- 10 oz of tomato sauce

AAAAAAAAAAAAAAAAAAAAAA

Methods:

A. In a pan, sauté the oregano and cloves in oil. Cooking the herbs and spices in oil helps to release their flavors and aromas, adding depth to the sauce.

B. Cook and stir the mixture for about 2 minutes. This step allows the oregano and cloves to infuse their flavors into the oil.

C. Add the tomato sauce, pepper, salt, and cooked spaghetti to the pan. Toss everything well to coat the spaghetti with the flavorful tomato sauce.

D. Cook the spaghetti in the sauce for about 1 minute, ensuring that it is heated through and fully coated with the sauce.

E. Serve the Spag and Tomato Sauce with cheese on top. Grated Parmesan or Pecorino Romano are popular choices for adding a savory and salty touch to the dish.

Cooking Notes:

A. To make the dish more robust and flavorful, you can add minced garlic and finely chopped onions along with the oregano and cloves in step 1. Sauté them until softened before adding the sauce and other ingredients.

B. For the tomato sauce, you can use store-bought marinara or homemade tomato sauce. If using store-bought, choose a high-quality sauce with your preferred level of seasoning.

C. You can also add other herbs and seasonings to the sauce, such as basil, thyme, or red pepper flakes, depending on your taste preferences.

D. If the sauce seems too thick, you can add a splash of pasta water or vegetable broth to achieve your desired consistency.

E. To enhance the flavor of the dish, consider adding cooked and sliced Italian sausage, cooked ground beef, or grilled chicken. These protein additions complement the tomato sauce and spaghetti well.

F. Al Dente Pasta: Cook the spaghetti until it is "al dente," which means it should be cooked to be firm to the bite. To achieve this, follow the package instructions for cooking time or taste test the pasta a minute or two before the recommended time. Overcooking the pasta will result in a mushy texture.

G. Fresh vs. Dried Oregano: You can use either fresh or dried oregano for this recipe. If using fresh oregano, add it towards the end of sautéing the herbs and spices, as it can lose its flavor if cooked for too long. For dried oregano, add it at the beginning to infuse the oil with its flavor.

H. Wine or Broth: For a richer and more complex flavor, you can deglaze the pan with a splash of red or white wine after sautéing the oregano and cloves. Let the wine simmer for a minute to cook off the alcohol. If you prefer a non-alcoholic option, vegetable or chicken broth can also be used.

I.   Tomato Paste: To intensify the tomato flavor, consider adding a tablespoon of tomato paste to the sauce before adding the tomato sauce. Tomato paste is concentrated and adds depth to the sauce.

J.   Fresh Tomatoes: If you have ripe fresh tomatoes, you can use them instead of tomato sauce. Chop the tomatoes and cook them down in the pan until they release their juices and form a thick sauce.

K.   Meatless Option: For a vegetarian version, omit the oregano and cloves and sauté minced garlic and onions in the oil. Proceed with adding the tomato sauce and seasonings. You can also add sautéed mushrooms or grilled eggplant for added texture and flavor.

L.   Using Reserved Pasta Water: Before draining the cooked spaghetti, reserve a cup of the pasta cooking water. If the sauce is too thick or needs more liquid, you can add a small amount of the pasta water to achieve the desired consistency.

M.   Leftovers: Spag and Tomato Sauce is a dish that reheats well, making it a great option for leftovers. Store any unused portions in an airtight container in the refrigerator for up to 3 days. Reheat gently in a pan or microwave, adding a splash of water or broth to refresh the sauce.

N.   Garnish Options: Besides grated cheese and fresh herbs, consider adding a drizzle of high-quality extra virgin olive oil or a sprinkle of red pepper flakes for added flavor and presentation.

O.   Family-Friendly: If serving to kids or those sensitive to spices, you can skip the cloves or use a smaller amount. Adjust the seasoning according to your family's taste preferences.

P.   Spag and Tomato Sauce is a classic comfort dish that allows for creativity and personalization. Feel free to experiment with different herbs, seasonings, and protein additions to create your ideal spaghetti dish. Enjoy this comforting and timeless meal with family and friends!

23. Salmon Stir Fry

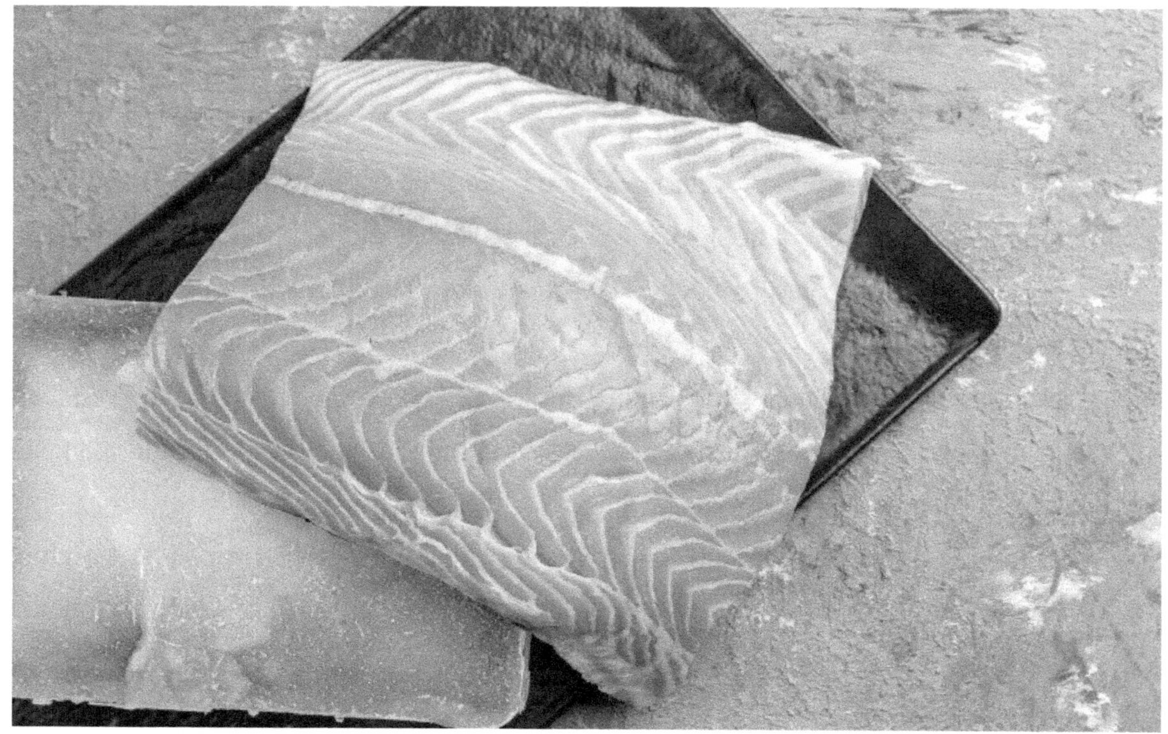

Salmon lovers, want to check this out?

Preparation Time: 05 Minutes

Cook Time: 10 Minutes

Serve: 2

List of Ingredients:

- 1 handful of toasted sesame seeds
- 2 garlic cloves
- 4 tbsp of soy sauce
- 1 tbsp of rice vinegar (seasoned)
- 1 tbsp of olive oil
- 1 pinch of powder ginger
- 1 tbsp of sesame oil
- 2 cups of chopped mushroom, broccolini, capsicum, and green peas
- 1 pound of chunked salmon filets

AAAAAAAAAAAAAAAAAAAAAAA

Methods:

A. In a wok, sauté the ginger and garlic in both oils. The combination of regular oil and sesame oil adds depth to the flavor profile of the dish.

B. Stir the ginger and garlic for about 2 minutes until they become fragrant. This step helps to release their aromas and infuse the oil with their flavors.

C. Add the salmon to the wok and cook for approximately 3 minutes, stirring occasionally. The salmon should be cooked through but still tender and moist.

D. Introduce the vegetables, sauce, and vinegar to the wok. The vegetables can be a mix of your choice, such as bell peppers, broccoli, carrots, snap peas, or baby corn. The sauce can be a combination of soy sauce, oyster sauce, or any other stir-fry sauce you prefer.

E. Continue to cook for another 3 minutes, allowing the flavors to meld together and the vegetables to become tender-crisp. Adjust the cooking time based on your desired level of crunchiness for the vegetables.

F. Serve the Salmon Stir Fry with rice to make it a complete and satisfying meal. Garnish with sesame seeds for added texture and nutty flavor.

Cooking Notes:

A. When cooking the salmon, make sure not to overcook it, as it can become dry and tough. Cook it just until it flakes easily with a fork, and it will remain juicy and flavorful.

B. To prevent the garlic and ginger from burning, stir them constantly while sautéing. Lower the heat if necessary to avoid excessive browning.

C. You can marinate the salmon in a mixture of soy sauce, garlic, and ginger before stir-frying to add even more flavor to the dish.

D. Feel free to add other vegetables or ingredients like mushrooms, onions, or baby corn to the stir-fry according to your taste preferences.

E. For some extra heat and a hint of spice, you can add a small amount of chili flakes or sliced red chili to the stir-fry.

F. If you prefer a thicker sauce, you can mix a tablespoon of cornstarch with water and add it to the stir-fry, allowing it to thicken slightly.

G. Resting the Salmon: For an even juicier and flavorful salmon, let it rest for a few minutes before slicing and adding it to the stir-fry. Resting allows the salmon's juices to redistribute and ensures a tender and moist texture.

H. Wok or High Heat Pan: A wok is ideal for stir-frying due to its shape and high heat conductivity. However, if you don't have a wok, you can use a high-heat pan or skillet. Just make sure it is large enough to accommodate all the ingredients without overcrowding, as overcrowding can lead to steaming instead of stir-frying.

I. Stir-Fry Order: When stir-frying with different vegetables, start with the harder and denser vegetables, such as carrots and broccoli, as they require more cooking time.

Add the softer vegetables, like bell peppers and snap peas, towards the end to retain their crispiness.

J. Flavorful Marinade: To enhance the salmon's taste, marinate it for about 15-30 minutes in a mixture of soy sauce, sesame oil, garlic, and ginger before cooking. This step not only adds flavor but also tenderizes the fish.

K. Doneness of Vegetables: The cooking time for vegetables can vary based on their size and thickness. To test their doneness, try a piece of each vegetable to ensure they are cooked to your liking. They should be tender-crisp with vibrant colors.

L. Sauce Adjustments: The sauce plays a crucial role in the overall flavor of the stir-fry. Feel free to adjust the amount of sauce, sweetness, or saltiness to suit your taste preferences. You can also add a splash of chicken or vegetable broth if you prefer a saucier dish.

M. Serving Suggestions: While serving with rice is a classic option, you can also enjoy the Salmon Stir Fry over noodles, quinoa, or cauliflower rice for a low-carb alternative. The stir-fry can also be served on its own as a light and healthy meal.

N. Leftovers: This dish is great for meal prep, and any leftovers can be stored in an airtight container in the refrigerator for up to 3 days. Reheat gently in a pan or microwave, adding a splash of water or broth to maintain moisture.

O. Nutritional Boost: Consider adding a handful of baby spinach or kale to the stir-fry during the last minute of cooking. This adds extra nutrients and vibrant green color to the dish.

P. Family-Friendly: If you're serving this stir-fry to kids or those who prefer milder flavors, reduce the amount of ginger or garlic. You can also serve some chili sauce or sriracha on the side for those who enjoy a spicier kick.

Q. Stir-fries are incredibly versatile and allow you to play with flavors and textures. Embrace creativity and experiment with different combinations of vegetables, sauces, and seasonings to create your perfect Salmon Stir Fry. Enjoy the delicious harmony of flavors and textures in this wholesome and satisfying meal!

24. Ginger Green Juice

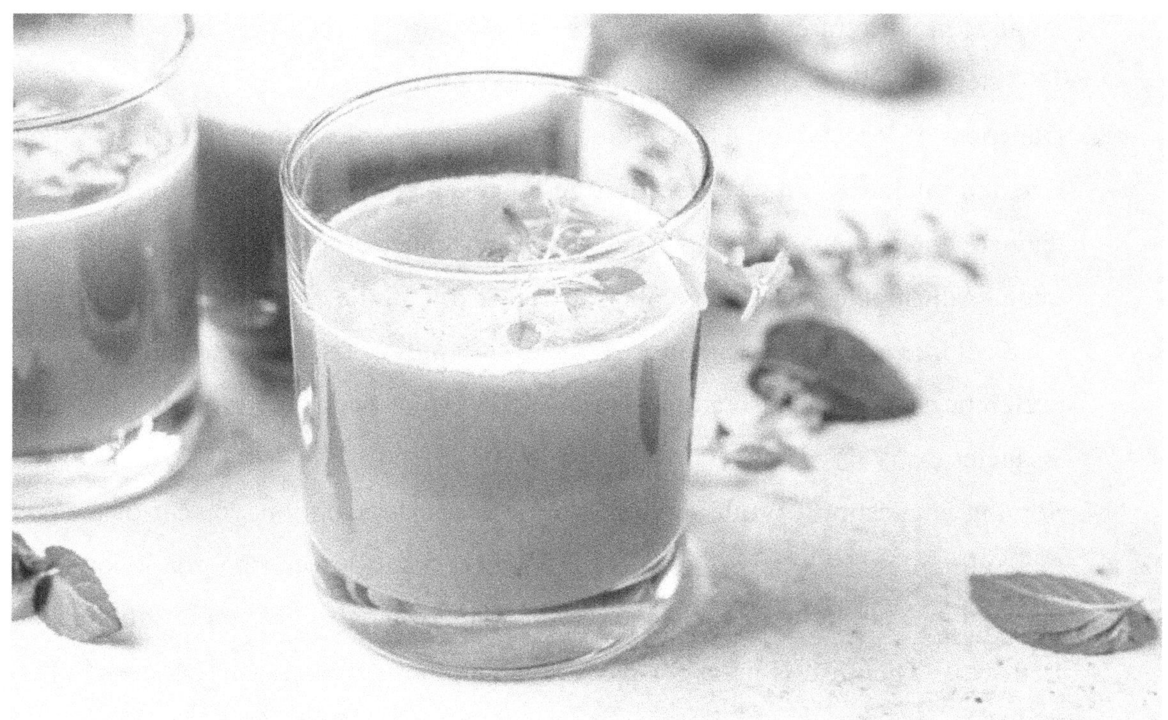

It's zingy and delicious!!

Preparation Time: 03 Minutes

Cook Time: Nil

Serve: 1

List of Ingredients:

- 2 chopped cored apples
- 1 chopped ginger finger
- 3 tbsp of lemon juice
- 1 chopped medium-sized cucumber
- 1 bunch of chopped kale

AAAAAAAAAAAAAAAAAAAAAA

Methods:

A. Prepare all the ingredients by chopping the cored apples, ginger finger, medium-sized cucumber, and kale. The ginger finger can be adjusted according to your preference for the level of spiciness.

B. Place all the chopped ingredients in a juicer or food processor. If you're using a juicer, you may need to cut the ingredients into smaller pieces to fit through the chute.

C. Add 3 tablespoons of lemon juice to the juicer or food processor. Lemon juice adds a tangy flavor and helps balance the sweetness of the apples.

D. Process or juice all the ingredients together until you get a smooth and well-blended consistency. Depending on the type of equipment you use, you may need to do this in batches.

E. Once the juice is ready, serve it immediately. Ginger Green Juice is best enjoyed fresh to retain its nutritional value and vibrant flavor.

Cooking Notes:

A. For a milder taste, you can peel the ginger before chopping it. This will reduce the intensity of the ginger flavor in the juice.

B. Feel free to adjust the ingredients according to your taste preferences. If you prefer a sweeter juice, you can add more apples. On the other hand, if you want a stronger ginger flavor, you can add more ginger.

C. You can strain the juice through a fine mesh strainer or cheesecloth to remove any pulp or fiber, but it's not necessary. Leaving the pulp in the juice adds extra fiber and nutrients.

D. If you don't have a juicer or a food processor, you can also use a blender to make the juice. However, you may need to add some water to help blend the ingredients smoothly.

E. Time-Saving Tip: To save time on busy mornings, you can prepare the ingredients in advance and store them in an airtight container in the refrigerator. This way, you can quickly assemble and juice the ingredients whenever you want a fresh glass of Ginger Green Juice.

F. Hydration Boost: If you prefer a lighter and more hydrating juice, you can add a splash of coconut water or filtered water to the ingredients before processing. This will dilute the juice slightly and make it even more refreshing.

G. Optional Additions: Customize the juice by adding other ingredients that you enjoy. For a citrusy twist, you can add a peeled and segmented orange or a splash of orange juice. Additionally, a small piece of fresh turmeric can complement the ginger's spiciness and provide additional health benefits.

H. Nut Butter or Seeds: For an extra dose of healthy fats and protein, consider adding a tablespoon of almond butter, chia seeds, or flaxseeds to the juice. These additions will help make the juice more filling and keep you energized throughout the day.

I. Ginger Preservation: If you buy ginger in larger quantities and want to keep it fresh, you can store it in the freezer. Simply peel the ginger, chop it into smaller pieces, and place them in a sealed freezer-safe bag. This way, you'll always have ginger on hand for your daily juice.

J. Glass Presentation: To elevate the presentation of your Ginger Green Juice, serve it in a tall glass with a sprig of fresh mint or a slice of cucumber as a garnish. This adds a touch of elegance and makes the juice even more appealing.

K. Reusing Pulp: Instead of discarding the leftover pulp after juicing, consider repurposing it in other recipes. The pulp can be added to smoothies, used in baking muffins or pancakes, or mixed into vegetable soups for added fiber and nutrition.

L. Juicing Greens: When using kale in the juicer, alternate the kale leaves with other juicer-friendly ingredients like cucumber or apple. This helps prevent the juicer from getting clogged and ensures a smoother juicing process.

M. Ginger Green Juice is a fantastic way to kickstart your day with a burst of nutrients and natural energy. Experiment with the ingredients and proportions to find the perfect balance of flavors and create a juice that suits your taste preferences. Enjoy this revitalizing and healthful beverage as a daily routine or a refreshing pick-me-up at any time of the day.

25. Honeydew Mint Smoothie

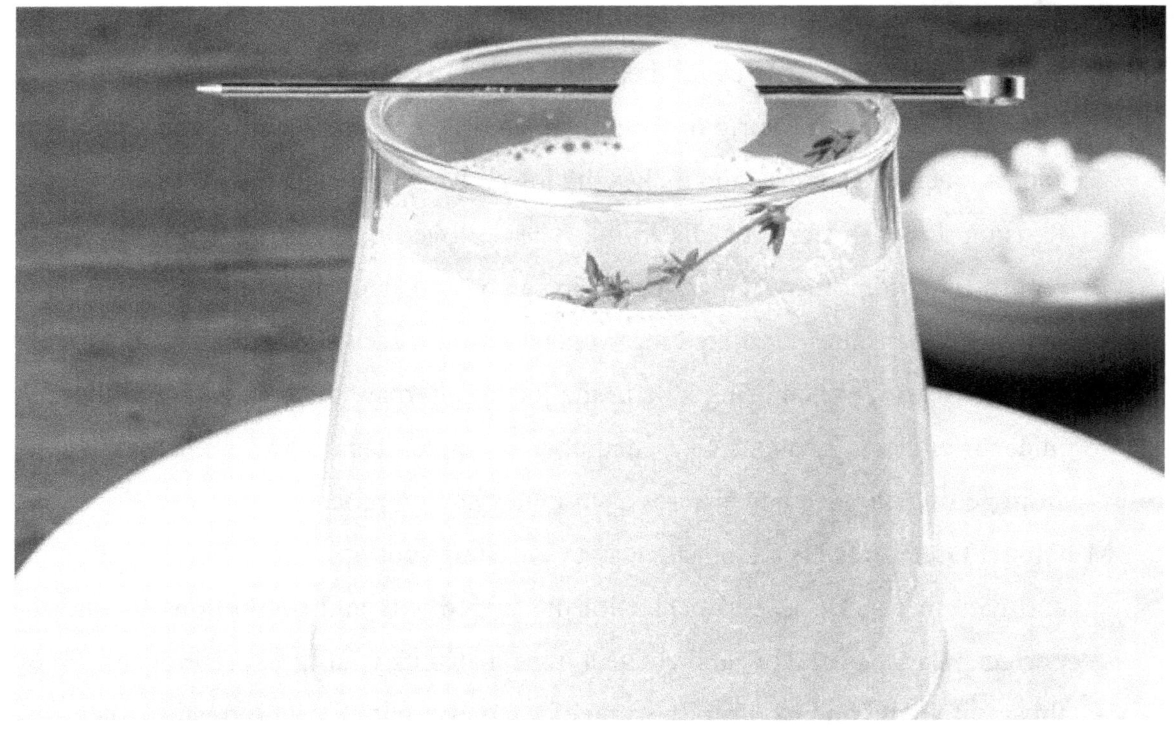

Well!!! Who knew a smoothie could be healthy and indulgent too?!

Preparation Time: 04 Minutes

Cook Time: Nil

Serve: 2

List of Ingredients:

- 1 mint leaf
- 2 cups of peeled and seeded honeydew melon (chopped)
- 1 tbsp of lemon juice
- 4 tbsp of coconut milk
- 1 tbsp of coconut nectar
- 1 cup of ice cubes

AAAAAAAAAAAAAAAAAAAAAA

Methods:

A. In a blender, combine the chopped honeydew melon, mint leaf, lemon juice, coconut milk, coconut nectar, and ice cubes.
B. Blend all the ingredients together until you get a smooth and creamy texture.
C. Pour the honeydew mint smoothie into glasses.
D. Garnish each glass with additional fresh mint leaves for an extra burst of flavor and a beautiful presentation.
E. Serve the refreshing honeydew mint smoothie immediately and enjoy its cool and invigorating taste.

Cooking Notes:

A. Make sure to use ripe and sweet honeydew melon for the best flavor in your smoothie.

B. Adjust the sweetness by adding more or less coconut nectar according to your taste preferences.

C. Mint Infusion: To infuse the smoothie with a stronger mint flavor, you can steep the fresh mint leaves in the coconut milk before blending. Heat the coconut milk until it's just about to simmer, then remove it from heat and add the mint leaves. Let them steep for a few minutes, then strain the coconut milk to remove the leaves. Use this infused coconut milk in the smoothie for an extra minty kick.

D. Pre-Chill Ingredients: For an even more refreshing experience, consider chilling the honeydew melon and coconut milk in the refrigerator before blending. This will give your smoothie an icy cold temperature without the need for additional ice cubes.

E. Sweetener Alternatives: If you prefer a different sweetener or want to keep it sugar-free, you can replace the coconut nectar with honey, agave syrup, maple syrup, or your preferred sweetener.

F. Garnish with Fruit: Elevate the presentation by garnishing the smoothie with thin slices of honeydew melon or other fresh fruits like berries or kiwi. These colorful additions add visual appeal and make the smoothie even more enticing.

G. Nutritional Boost: To boost the nutritional content of the smoothie, consider adding a handful of fresh spinach or kale. The mild flavor of the honeydew melon and mint can easily mask the greens, providing an extra nutrient punch.

H. Coconut Water: If you want a lighter flavor profile, you can replace some or all of the coconut milk with coconut water. This variation will result in a more hydrating and less creamy smoothie.

I. Non-Dairy Options: For a vegan or dairy-free version, use non-dairy milk alternatives like almond milk, oat milk, or soy milk instead of coconut milk.

J. Protein Boost: To turn this refreshing drink into a satisfying breakfast or post-workout option, you can add a scoop of protein powder, Greek yogurt, or silken tofu. This addition will provide a boost of protein and make the smoothie more filling.

K. Make-Ahead and Storage: If you have leftover smoothie, store it in a sealed container in the refrigerator for up to 24 hours. Before serving, give it a quick shake or stir, as separation may occur over time.

L. The honeydew mint smoothie is a fantastic way to cool off and indulge in the delightful flavors of honeydew and mint. Experiment with the ingredients to suit your taste, and enjoy this refreshing drink as a healthy and hydrating treat on warm days or any time you crave a revitalizing beverage.

26. 4 Ingredients: Fall Juice

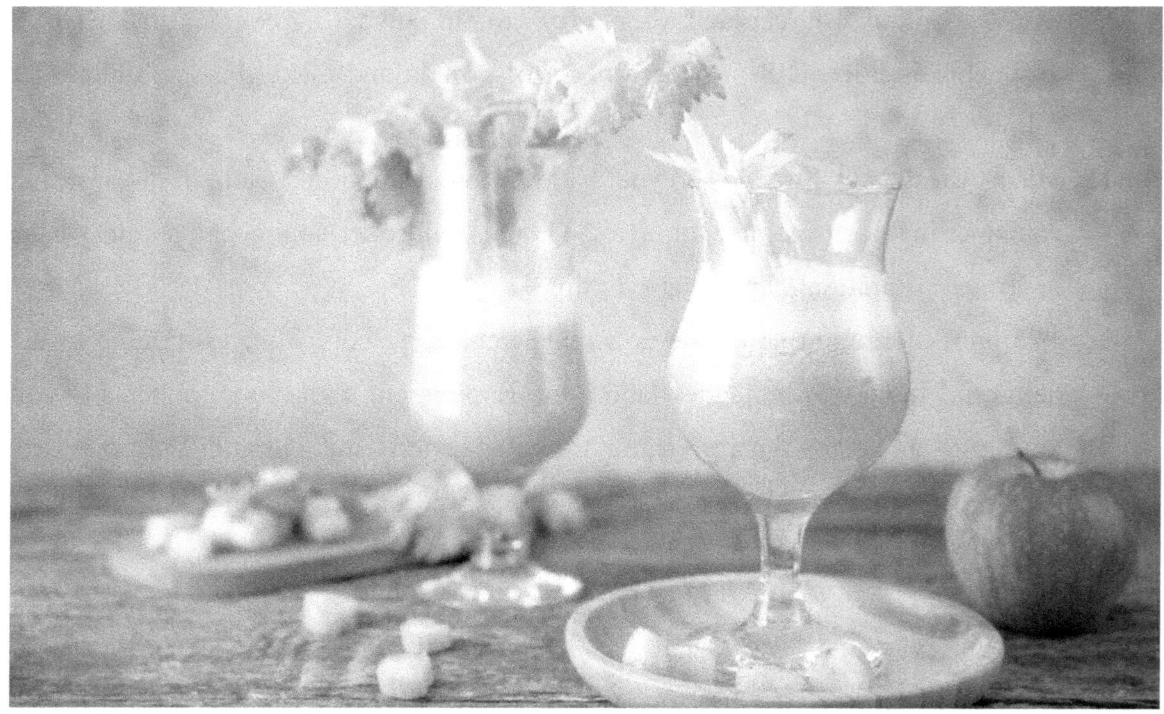

Ever thought of adding Swiss Chard to your smoothies?

This is an opportunity to try it out!!

Preparation Time: 03 Minutes

Cook Time: Nil

Serve: 1

List of Ingredients:

- 1 celery stick
- 2 cups of Swiss chard
- 1 orange (peeled and seeded)
- 5 chopped apples

AAAAAAAAAAAAAAAAAAAAAA

Methods:

A. Wash and prepare the celery stick, Swiss chard, orange, and apples. Remove any seeds from the orange and core the apples.

B. Chop the celery, Swiss chard, orange, and apples into smaller pieces to fit into the juicer chute easily.

C. Add all the prepared ingredients to the juicer. Make sure to layer them evenly to ensure efficient juicing.

D. Turn on the juicer and juice all the ingredients until you extract all the liquids from the celery, Swiss chard, orange, and apples.

E. Once the juicing process is complete, give the juice a quick stir to mix all the flavors.

F. Pour the fall juice into a glass and serve immediately.

Cooking Notes:

A. To get the most out of your juicer, make sure to use fresh and ripe produce.

B. If you prefer a sweeter juice, you can add a touch of honey or maple syrup to enhance the natural sweetness of the apples and oranges.

C. Greens and Bitterness: Swiss chard can sometimes have a slightly bitter taste. If you prefer a milder juice, you can blanch the Swiss chard before juicing it. Boil it in water for a minute or two, then immediately transfer it to ice water to preserve its vibrant color and reduce bitterness.

D. Temperature and Chill: If you prefer a refreshing and chilled fall juice, you can refrigerate the celery, Swiss chard, and apples before juicing. Chilling the ingredients will result in a cooler and more enjoyable juice.

E. Pulp Utilization: Don't discard the leftover pulp from the juicing process! You can use it creatively in other recipes, such as adding it to soups, stews, or muffins for added fiber and nutrients.

F. Nutritional Boost: For an added nutritional boost, consider incorporating other nutrient-rich ingredients into the juice. Kale, spinach, cucumber, and ginger are excellent choices that can enhance the nutritional content of your fall juice.

G. Juice Separation: Natural separation of the juice may occur over time due to the varying densities of the ingredients. If this happens, give the juice a gentle shake or stir before serving to remix the flavors.

H. Reusing Pulp: If you don't have immediate plans to use the pulp, you can compost it or freeze it for future use. The frozen pulp can be used as a base for smoothies or added to sauces and dressings.

I. Variety of Apples: Experiment with different apple varieties to find the one that best suits your taste preferences. Sweeter apples like Honeycrisp or Fuji can provide a delightful sweetness to the juice, while tart apples like Granny Smith can add a tangy flavor.

J. Freshly Squeezed Orange Juice: If you don't have a juicer, you can manually squeeze the orange to extract the juice. Freshly squeezed orange juice adds a vibrant citrus flavor to the fall juice.

K. Hydration: Drinking fall juice can be a great way to stay hydrated, especially during the cooler months when we may forget to drink enough water.

L. Fall juice is a refreshing and nutritious beverage that celebrates the flavors of the season. Whether you enjoy it as a quick pick-me-up or a part of your daily routine, this juice provides a medley of vitamins, minerals, and antioxidants. Feel free to customize the recipe to your liking and enjoy the wholesome goodness of fresh, homemade juice!

27. Orecchiette and Cavolo Nero

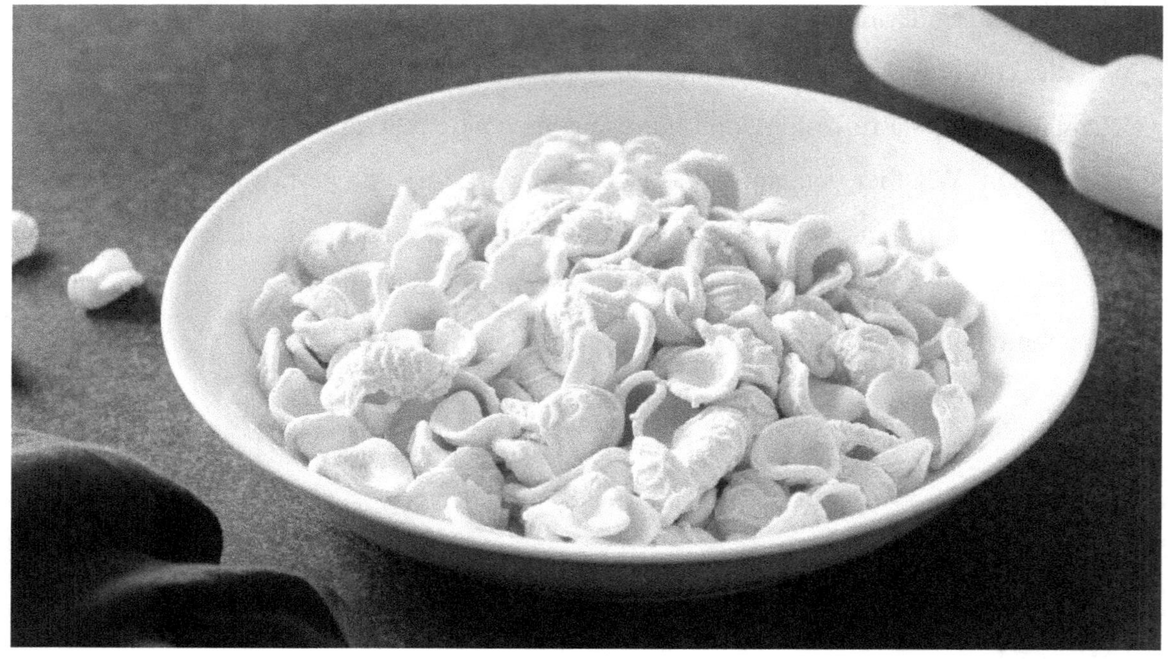

Don't let the strange name fool you; it is just Tuscan pasta and exotic veggie delicacy!!!

Preparation Time: 05 Minutes

Cook Time: 10 Minutes

Serve: 2

List of Ingredients:

- 250g of cooked orecchiette pasta (drained with 6 tbsp water reserved)
- 1 chopped seeded red chili
- 1 handful of grated Parmesan cheese
- 2 anchovy filets
- 70g of olive oil
- 1 chopped garlic clove
- 1 tbsp of salt
- 2 handfuls of blanched and rinsed cavolo nero (chopped)
- 1 tbsp of pepper

AAAAAAAAAAAAAAAAAAAAAAA

Methods:

A. In a pan with oil, sauté the anchovies, chili, and garlic for about 3 minutes. This step helps to infuse the oil with the flavors of the anchovies and spices.

B. Add the Cavolo Nero (also known as Lacinato kale or Tuscan kale) to the pan. Cook and stir for an additional 2 minutes. The Cavolo Nero will wilt slightly and absorb the flavors from the anchovies and garlic.

C. Cook the orecchiette pasta according to package instructions until al dente. Before draining the pasta, reserve a cup of the pasta cooking water.

D. Add the cooked orecchiette pasta to the pan with Cavolo Nero and toss well to combine. The pasta will absorb the flavors of the sautéed ingredients.

E. Pour in the reserved pasta cooking water to create a light sauce that coats the pasta and greens. The starchy pasta water helps to bind the flavors together and gives the dish a silky texture.

F. Season with freshly ground black pepper and salt to taste. Be cautious with the salt as the anchovies are already salty.

G. Serve the Orecchiette and Cavolo Nero in a large serving dish. Garnish with grated cheese of your choice, such as Pecorino Romano or Parmesan.

Cooking Notes:

A. Orecchiette is a type of pasta with a cup-like shape that is perfect for holding the Cavolo Nero and sauce.

B. Cavolo Nero is a dark leafy green that has a slightly bitter taste. If you can't find Cavolo Nero, you can use regular kale or even spinach as a substitute.

C. Anchovies add a savory umami flavor to the dish. If you prefer a vegetarian option, you can omit the anchovies or replace them with capers for a similar briny taste.

D. Adjust the level of chili according to your spice preference. You can use fresh chili or red pepper flakes for a milder or spicier version.

E. Toasting the Anchovies: For an intensified flavor, you can toast the anchovies in the pan for a minute or two before adding the garlic and chili. This step enhances the umami taste of the anchovies and creates a more complex sauce.

F. Adding Lemon Zest: To brighten up the dish and balance the flavors, consider adding some freshly grated lemon zest before serving. The zest adds a citrusy note that complements the bitterness of the Cavolo Nero.

G. Using Whole Garlic Cloves: Instead of minced garlic, you can use whole garlic cloves that are slightly smashed to release their aroma. Remove the cloves before serving, or leave them in if you enjoy the stronger garlic flavor.

H. Cooking the Greens Separately: To preserve the vibrant green color of the Cavolo Nero, you can blanch or steam the greens separately before adding them to the sautéed anchovies and garlic. This helps retain their color and nutrients.

I. Cooking with White Wine: For an extra layer of flavor, deglaze the pan with a splash of white wine after sautéing the anchovies, chili, and garlic. Allow the alcohol to evaporate before adding the Cavolo Nero.

J. Experimenting with Additional Ingredients: This recipe provides a wonderful base for experimentation. You can add sun-dried tomatoes, roasted pine nuts, or olives for added texture and flavor.

K. Making it Creamy: If you prefer a creamier dish, stir in a tablespoon of cream or a dollop of mascarpone cheese just before serving.

L. Grating the Cheese Finely: For better cheese distribution and smoother melting, grate the cheese finely before sprinkling it over the pasta.

M. Serving Suggestions: For a complete meal, serve the Orecchiette and Cavolo Nero with a fresh green salad or garlic bread on the side.

N. Orecchiette and Cavolo Nero is a delightful Italian-inspired pasta dish that brings together the rich umami of anchovies with the earthy bitterness of Cavolo Nero. With its simple preparation and satisfying flavors, it's an excellent choice for a quick and flavorful weeknight dinner. Enjoy the delicious combination of pasta, greens, and savory anchovies!

28. Mexican Rice and Chicken

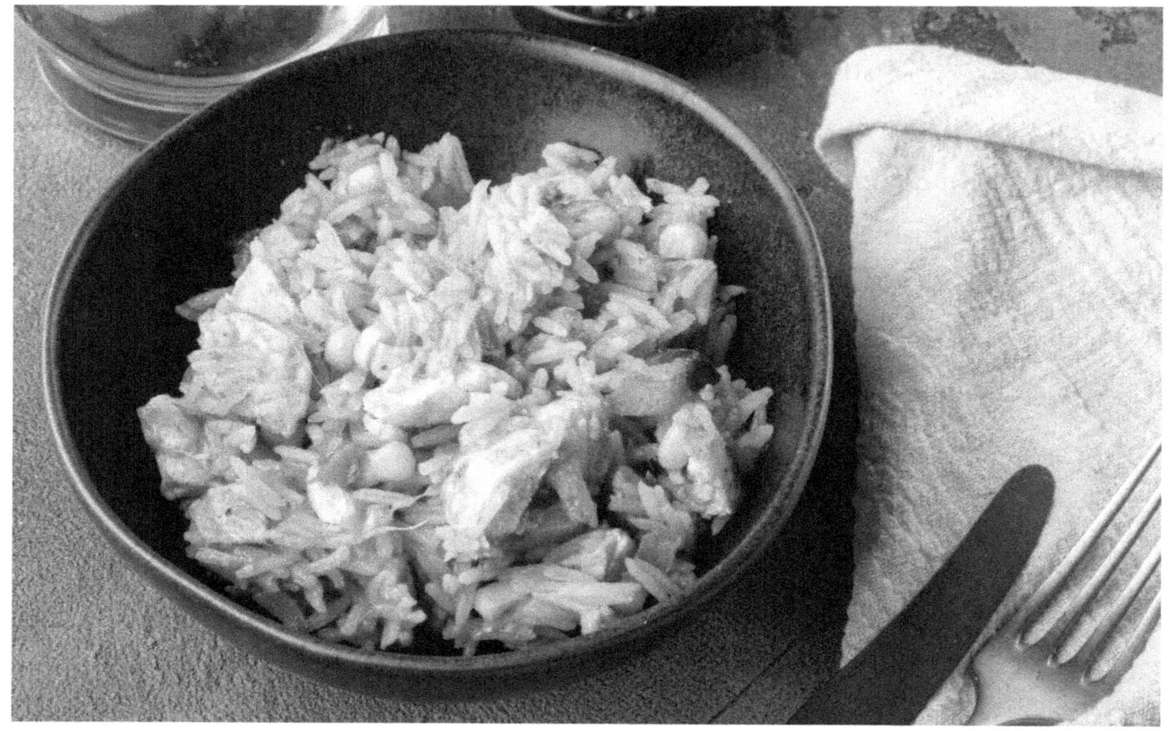

Let's take a trip down to Mexico!!!!

Preparation Time:08 Minutes

Cook Time: 20 Minutes

Serve:3

List of Ingredients:

- 1 tbsp of salt
- 1 lb. of cubed lean chicken breast
- 2 oz of green chilies
- 10 oz of tomato sauce
- 1 pinch of cumin
- 1 pinch of chili powder
- 1 cup of chicken broth
- 1 pinch of pepper
- 1 diced onion
- 1 tbsp of oil
- 1 cup of raw white rice (long grain)
- 1 tsp of garlic powder

AAAAAAAAAAAAAAAAAAAAAA

Methods:

A. In a pan with oil, sauté the onions for about 3 minutes until they become translucent and aromatic.

B. Add the chicken, diced bell pepper, minced garlic, salt, chili powder, and cumin to the pan. Cook for about 7 minutes until the chicken is browned and cooked through.

C. Stir in the rice and toast it for about 4 minutes. Toasting the rice enhances its nutty flavor and prevents it from becoming too mushy when cooked.

D. Pour in the chicken broth, diced green chilies, and tomato sauce. The chicken broth adds moisture and flavor to the rice, while the diced green chilies and tomato sauce provide a mild spicy kick and tanginess.

E. Bring the mixture to a boil, then reduce the heat to low. Cover the pan and let the rice simmer until it is fully cooked and has absorbed all the liquid. This usually takes about 15-20 minutes, but it may vary depending on the type of rice used.

F. Once the rice is done, fluff it with a fork and taste for seasoning. Adjust the salt and spices if needed.

G. Serve the Mexican rice and chicken in a large serving dish, garnished with fresh chopped cilantro. The cilantro adds a refreshing herbal flavor that compliments the dish well.

Cooking Notes:

A. You can use long-grain white rice or medium-grain rice for this recipe. If using brown rice, the cooking time may be longer, and you may need to add a bit more liquid.

B. For a spicier version, you can add diced jalapenos or a pinch of cayenne pepper along with the other spices.

C. Resting the Chicken: For more flavorful and tender chicken, you can marinate the chicken in a mixture of lime juice, olive oil, and Mexican spices for 30 minutes to an hour before cooking. This step adds extra depth of flavor to the dish.

D. Customizing the Spices: Mexican cuisine is known for its bold and vibrant flavors. Feel free to experiment with additional spices such as paprika, oregano, coriander, or even a pinch of cinnamon to create your unique flavor profile.

E. Using Fresh or Canned Tomatoes: While tomato sauce provides a smooth texture, you can also use diced fresh tomatoes or canned diced tomatoes for a chunkier texture. If using fresh tomatoes, sauté them with the chicken until they soften before adding the rice.

F. Cooking the Rice Separately: To prevent the rice from becoming too mushy, you can cook it separately and then mix it with the chicken and vegetable mixture. This method allows you to control the texture of the rice more precisely.

G. Incorporating Black Beans: For added protein and a more authentic Mexican touch, consider adding black beans to the dish. Canned black beans can be rinsed and added along with the chicken broth.

H. Using Saffron: For a luxurious twist, you can infuse the rice with a pinch of saffron threads. Soak the saffron in a tablespoon of warm water before adding it to the rice, and enjoy the beautiful golden hue and aromatic flavor.

I. Keeping it Mild or Extra Spicy: Adjust the amount of chili powder and green chilies according to your spice tolerance. If serving for a crowd with varying spice preferences, you can offer hot sauce on the side for individuals to add as they desire.

J. Make-Ahead and Storage: This dish can be made ahead and refrigerated for up to 3 days. Reheat it in the microwave or on the stovetop with a splash of water or broth to refresh the flavors.

K. Adapting for the Instant Pot or Rice Cooker: You can adapt this recipe for the Instant Pot or a rice cooker. Sauté the onions, garlic, chicken, and spices using the "Sauté" function of the Instant Pot. Then add the rice, broth, green chilies, and tomato sauce, and pressure cook according to your rice cooker's instructions or Instant Pot guidelines.

L. Mexican rice and chicken is a versatile and satisfying dish that is sure to please everyone at the table. By customizing the spices and adding your favorite ingredients, you can create a delicious one-pot meal that suits your taste perfectly. Enjoy the flavors of Mexico in the comfort of your home!

29. Rotelle Burrata, Spinach and Almonds

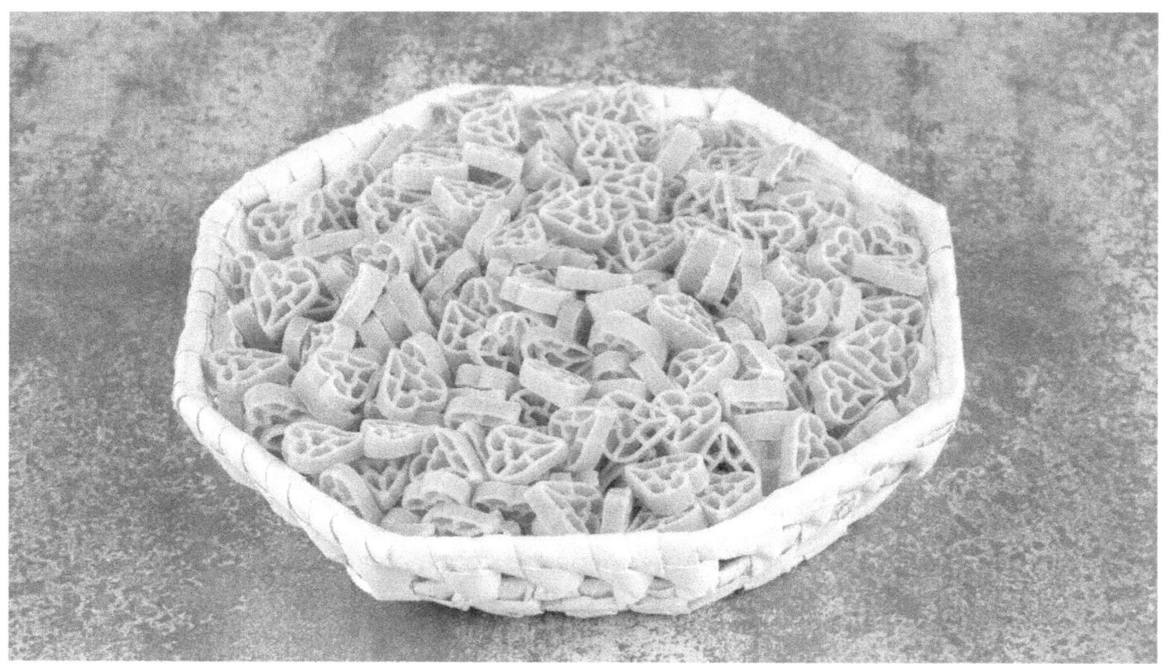

Do you actually want to indulge yourself in a light, delicious and healthy meal after a hard day's job? Then, you need to explore this delicacy!!

Preparation Time: 05 Minutes

Cook Time: 10 Minutes

Serve: 2

List of Ingredients:

- 50g of slivered almonds
- 1 chopped garlic clove
- 100g of shredded mozzarella
- 40 ml of canola oil
- 100g of chopped spinach leaves
- 1 handful of lemon zest
- 10g of butter
- 200g of cooked rotelle pasta
- 30 ml of lemon juice

AAAAAAAAAAAAAAAAAAAAAAA

Methods:

A. In a pan, melt the butter over medium heat. Add the almonds and minced garlic to the pan.

B. Cook the almonds and garlic in the melted butter for about 2 minutes, stirring occasionally. This helps release the flavors of the garlic and lightly toast the almonds.

C. Add the fresh spinach and rotelle pasta to the pan. Cook and stir everything together for about 4 minutes until the spinach wilts and the pasta is cooked to your desired doneness.

D. Once the pasta and spinach are cooked, remove the pan from heat.

E. Serve the Rotelle Burrata, Spinach, and Almonds pasta on a plate or in a bowl.

F. Garnish the dish with lemon zest and a squeeze of lemon juice to add a bright and refreshing flavor to the pasta.

G. Serve the pasta with burrata cheese and breadcrumbs on top. The creamy burrata cheese adds richness to the dish, and the breadcrumbs provide a nice crunchy texture.

Cooking Notes:

A. You can use any type of pasta you prefer, not just rotelle. Fusilli, penne, or farfalle would work well too.

B. Feel free to add other vegetables or protein to the dish. Sliced cherry tomatoes, grilled chicken, or sautéed mushrooms would be delicious additions.

C. Adjust the amount of garlic, lemon zest, and juice according to your taste preference.

D. To Toast the Almonds: For extra flavor and crunch, you can toast the almonds separately before adding them to the pan. Simply spread the almonds on a baking sheet and bake them in a preheated oven at 350°F (175°C) for about 5-7 minutes or until lightly golden. Keep an eye on them to prevent burning.

E. Blanch the Spinach: If you prefer a softer texture for the spinach, blanch it briefly before adding it to the pan. Bring a pot of salted water to a boil, and then quickly blanch the spinach for about 30 seconds. Immediately transfer it to a bowl of ice water to stop the cooking process. Drain the spinach and squeeze out any excess water before adding it to the pasta.

F. Cooking the Pasta Al Dente: Cooking the pasta to al dente, meaning it's firm but not too soft, is essential for this dish. Test the pasta a minute or two before the recommended cooking time on the package. It should have a slight bite to it as it will continue to cook slightly in the pan with the sauce.

G. Lemon Zest and Juice: The lemon zest adds a fragrant citrus aroma to the pasta, while the lemon juice brightens the flavors and balances the richness of the butter and cheese. Adjust the amount of zest and juice based on your preference for acidity.

H. Making the Breadcrumbs: To make the breadcrumbs, simply tear or chop stale bread into small pieces, then pulse them in a food processor until you get coarse crumbs. Toast the breadcrumbs in a dry pan over medium heat until they turn golden brown and crispy.

I. Optional Wine: For a more sophisticated flavor profile, you can deglaze the pan with a splash of dry white wine after cooking the garlic and almonds. Allow the wine to reduce slightly before adding the pasta and spinach to the pan.

J. Keeping it Vegetarian or Vegan: To make this dish vegetarian or vegan, use a plant-based butter substitute and omit the cheese or use a vegan alternative. There are vegan burrata options available that can mimic the creamy texture of traditional burrata.

K. Reheating: If you have leftovers, you can reheat the pasta gently in a pan with a splash of water or vegetable broth to prevent it from drying out.

L. Serving Suggestions: Serve the Rotelle Burrata, Spinach, and Almonds pasta with a simple green salad or a side of garlic bread for a complete and satisfying meal.

M. This Rotelle Burrata, Spinach, and Almonds pasta offers a delightful combination of flavors and textures. It's a versatile dish that can be easily customized to suit your taste preferences, making it a go-to recipe for a delicious and comforting meal.

30. Blueberry Mint Green Smoothie

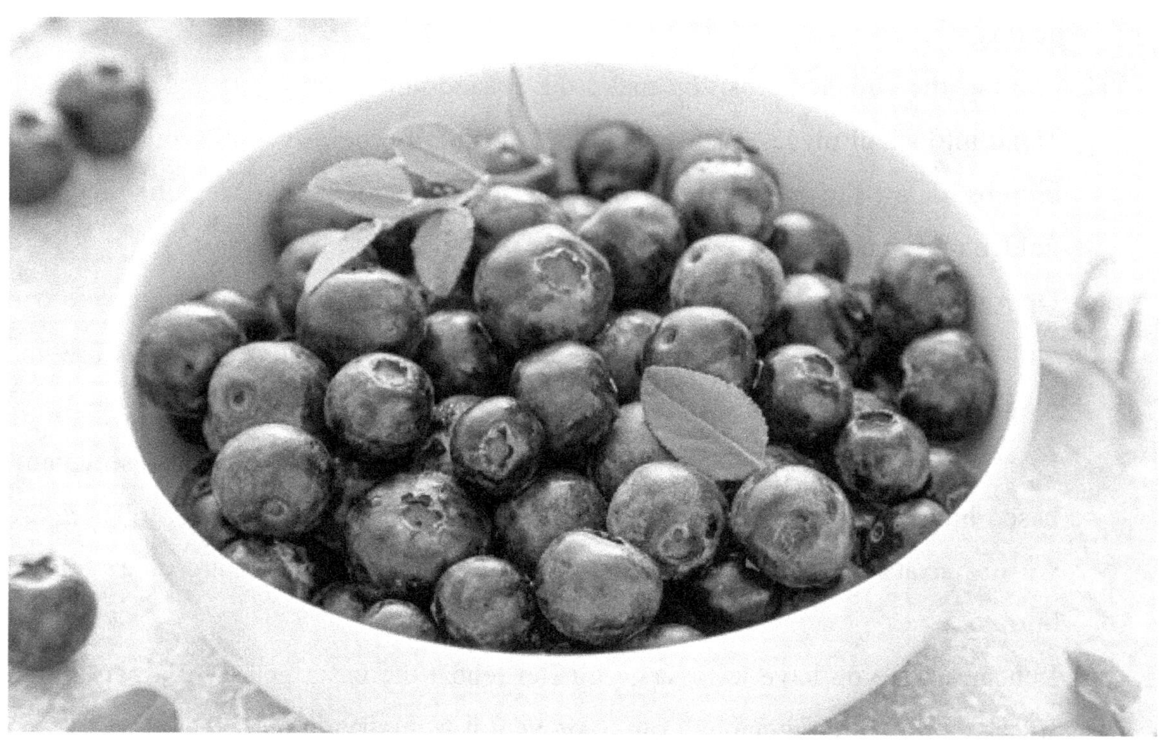

The combined taste of mint and blueberry gives this smoothie a delicious and unique flavor.

Preparation Time: 03 Minutes

Cook Time: Nil

Serve: 1

List of ingredients:

- 1 cup of blueberry
- 1 handful of ice
- 2 mint leaves
- 1 chopped kiwi
- 1 cup of spinach
- 8 tbsp of coconut water

AAAAAAAAAAAAAAAAAAAAAA

Methods:

A. Add the blueberries, ice, mint leaves, chopped kiwi, spinach, and coconut water to a blender or food processor.
B. Process the ingredients for about 3 minutes until everything is well blended and smooth. The smoothie should have a vibrant green color with specks of blueberries.
C. Pour the Blueberry Mint Green Smoothie into a glass and enjoy immediately.

Cooking Notes:

A. You can use fresh or frozen blueberries for this smoothie. If using frozen blueberries, you may need to adjust the amount of ice or coconut water to achieve the desired consistency.
B. Mint leaves add a refreshing flavor to the smoothie, but if you don't have mint on hand, you can skip it or substitute with a small amount of fresh basil or parsley for a different herbaceous twist.
C. Feel free to customize the smoothie to your taste. If you prefer it sweeter, you can add a drizzle of honey or a few drops of liquid stevia. Alternatively, if you want to boost the protein content, you can add a scoop of your favorite protein powder.

D. The kiwi adds natural sweetness and a subtle tang to the smoothie. You can leave the skin on the kiwi for added fiber and nutrients, or peel it if you prefer a smoother texture.

E. Greens Variations: While spinach is used in this recipe, you can experiment with other leafy greens, such as kale, Swiss chard, or arugula. Each green will add its unique flavor and nutritional benefits to the smoothie.

F. Prepping the Kiwi: When chopping the kiwi, you can cut it into small cubes or slices for easier blending. If your blender has difficulty blending the kiwi seeds, you can strain the smoothie through a fine mesh sieve before serving.

G. Boosting Nutrients: For an extra nutritional boost, you can add other superfood ingredients to the smoothie, such as chia seeds, flaxseeds, hemp seeds, or spirulina powder. These additions will provide extra fiber, omega-3 fatty acids, and protein.

H. Freezing the Ingredients: To save time and reduce the need for ice, you can freeze the blueberries and chopped kiwi in advance. Pre-freezing the fruits will result in a creamier and thicker smoothie without diluting the flavors with extra ice.

I. Creating Layers: To enhance the presentation and taste, consider creating layers in the smoothie. Blend the green layer (spinach, mint, coconut water) first and pour it into the glass. Then blend the blueberry layer (blueberries, kiwi, ice) separately and gently pour it on top of the green layer.

J. Adding Creaminess: If you prefer a creamier smoothie, you can add half of a ripe banana or a scoop of avocado to the blend. The banana or avocado will give the smoothie a rich and velvety texture.

K. Adjusting Sweetness: If you're using ripe and sweet blueberries and kiwi, you may not need any additional sweeteners. Taste the smoothie before adding honey or stevia to determine if it's sweet enough to your liking.

L. Prepping Ahead: To save time in the morning, you can prepare smoothie packs by pre-measuring the blueberries, chopped kiwi, and mint leaves in separate freezer bags. Store the packs in the freezer and simply blend them with the spinach and coconut water when you're ready to make the smoothie.

M. Serving Suggestions: Garnish the Blueberry Mint Green Smoothie with a sprig of fresh mint, a slice of kiwi, or a few blueberries for an elegant touch. Serving it in a chilled glass adds to the refreshing experience.

N. Making it Creamy and Dairy-Free: To make the smoothie creamier without using dairy, you can use coconut milk or almond milk instead of coconut water. This will give the smoothie a richer texture and enhance the coconut flavor.

O. Enjoy this vibrant and nutritious Blueberry Mint Green Smoothie as a refreshing and energizing beverage to kick-start your day or to enjoy as a healthy snack. Packed with goodness and bursting with flavors, it's a delightful way to incorporate more fruits and greens into your diet!

See You Again

Thank you for purchasing and reading my book. Your support means a lot, and I'm grateful you chose my book among many options. I write to help people like you, who appreciate every word.

Please share your thoughts on the book, as reader feedback helps me grow and improve. Your insights may even inspire others. Thanks again!

9 798864 717158